· List of Contributors ·

Dr. Marie Miczak, D.Sc., P.hD., CNC

Author of *Nature's Weeds, Native Medicine and How Not to Kill Yourself with Deadly Interactions*, she is a member of the American College of Clinical Pharmacology, certified nutritional consultant and professor at Brookdale College, Lincroft NJ. A frequent guest of both radio and television shows including NBC News, Dr. Miczak is internationally published in magazines and on the web, including at her official website www.miczak.com and click-on.to/apothecary. Contact Dr. Miczak toll free at 1-877-234-5350, ext. 676 or at miczak@juno.com.

Barbara M. Martin

Garden columnist Barbara M. Martin telecommutes as a professional horticulturist for the National Gardening Association and works in the south central Pennsylvania area as a garden designer and consultant specializing in herbs, perennials and historic gardens. With over twenty years practical experience she shares her love of gardening through lectures and classes for children and adults. You will find her writings on the Internet and in print. You may contact Barbara at martin@mail.cvn.net for immediate response.

Karyn Siegel-Maier

A writer for a number of magazines and websites on the topics of botanical medicine, nutrition and general health issues, she is also the author of *The Naturally Clean Home and 50 Simple Ways to Pamper Your Baby* both by Storey Books.

D0920054

How Flowers Heal

The Mind, Body & Soul

Marie Anakee Miczak

Writers Club Press
San Jose · New York · Lincoln · Shanghai

How Flowers Heal
The Mind, Body & Soul

ISBN: 0-595-09427-9

Published by Writers Club Press, an imprint of iUniverse.com, Inc.

For information address:
iUniverse.com, Inc.
620 North 48th Street
Suite 201
Lincoln, NE 68504-3467
www.iuniverse.com

URL: http://www.writersclub.com

· Dedication ·

I would like to dedicate this book to my wonderful brother Joe, who never complained about having to take over 200 slides, visitng all the botanical gardens with me and not getting paid. You're truly the best!

· Contents ·

· Acknowledgements ·

Firstly I would like to thank my brother Joe for sticking with me on this project! Second I would like to thank my dad, Joe Sr., for taking me to some wonderful botanical gardens around NJ. Third, I would like to thank my mother for also helping me so much in every area of this book, including going to gardens with me, writing the Native American Floral Use area and giving sage advice. Without her these books would not have been possible. I would also like to thank Barbara M. Martin and Karyn Siegel-Maier (fellow Suite101 Contributing Editors) for allowing me to reprint their wonderful articles. Also a big thank you to the countless people from all corners of the globe who contacted me with helpful information on flowers.

· Chronology ·

Other Titles by Marie Anakee Miczak include:
  Seceret Potions, Elixirs & Concoctions (Lotus Press)
  Mehndi (BBOTW)

· Introduction ·

When the word flower is mentioned in the context of healing, what is the first thought that comes to mind? For many, it is Aromatherapy or Bach Flower remedies. Still one should note all the other forms of natural medicine flowers are used in. The similarities in their healing effects tends to validate their traditional uses. In this book, you will be able to learn about the ways flowers have been used throughout history in healing and for pleasure. Likewise you will be able to cross reference charts and weigh the benefits against the precautions to make an educated decision to determine if a particular floral remedy is right for you. All botanicals, including flowers, can have side effects like prescription and OTC drugs and some should never be used if you are pregnant or suffer from a long term condition such as high blood pressure. It is always important to research as much as possible before using a floral botanical and to do a patch test before using a remedy. This book will also serve to show that one form of healing or botanical is not a *cure all*. Every culture has created their own form of healing to not only suit their particular needs, but to make use of the botanicals they have access to. It is unrealistic to think one culture or one form of healing holds all of the answers and is *the* only true form of healing. If this were the case, every geographic group of people without the knowledge of this one healing method would have perished long ago. In almost every part of the natural environment, there are remedies to be found if you look hard enough.

Aromatherapy vs. Aromacology

When many people think of the healing effect of flowers they envision Aromatherapy and the wonderful aromatic qualities of essential oils. This is quite understandable. Flowers growing in nature are many times highly aromatic. Unfortunately, due to mass commercialization, the true power of Aromatherapy has been confused with essence use and Aromacology. Back in the 80's and early 90's, when the American public and other countries, were first discovering the effects of essential oils, they were exposed to thinking that the main healing action of Aromatherapy was on a olfactory level. When the essential oils were sniffed, the molecules were carried through the nose and olfactory system which is said to be hard/soft wired to the brain. The healing effect would then be a result of the body being triggered to heal itself. Application of the essential oil was also discussed but because most of the clinical research had been done using essential oils on the olfactory system. Therefore this is what was emphasized as the healing power of Aromatherapy. Major perfume industries then saw a new way of marketing their fragrance oils and perfumes. They sought to blend the current conceptions about Aromatherapy's healing actions with their lab created scents and essences. They also saw Aromatherapy as a threat to their industry; more and more people were buying pure essential oils and creating their own personal scents instead of manufactured perfumes. In an effort to counter this, a new form of essence science was created called Aromacology, the study of scents on the olfactory system and it's relation to health and healing. Not fully understanding the difference between Aromatherapy and Aromacology, media outlets used information provided from those familiar with only Aromacology. This, of course, led to much confusion over the true healing qualities of essential oils. As years go by, more and more is being understood about the effects essential oils have when applied to the skin and how simply smelling a particular oil most likely will fail to produce any real improvement to a condition. Such is the case with burns and lavender essential oil. While "calming" and "antimicrobial" are both used to describe some of the actions of lavender, many are confused as to what to make of this information in the midst of the new Aromacology movement. Likewise, many believe one only needs to smell a fragrance or candle to benefit from the calming and antimicrobial actions. This thinking has also resulted in the misbelief that fragrance oils can be used in the same exact way as essential oils. While the calming effect of lavender is achieved through smell or on an Aromacology level, the antimicrobial actions occur when lavender is released into the air or applied to the skin. Fragrance oil of lavender "may" have the clarning effect but is unable to kill germs, aside from the alcohol used as a base. Fragrance oils and mock essences are like prescription drugs, only one or two components are recreated, most often the scent, from man made chemicals. Aromacology can be likened to western medicine, it doesn't allow for the true holistic treatment of the mind, body and soul as a whole. Classical Aromatherapy on the other hand is a true holistic form of healing. Each essential oil when administered takes into consideration ones psychological state and physical state, healing both simultaneously. Aromacology has it's place but it shouldn't be taken over Aromatherapy, as essential oil use is literally thousands of years old while fragrance oils have only been in production since the 1950's and has shown highly unpredictable results on healing people. A fine example of this is the huge failure of a citrus scented pen like device that would be held under the nose in attempt to make one lose weight and stop craving junk food. A small number of people favorably reacted to the essence for a while but the majority didn't notice any results at all. While certain citrus essential oils, such as grapefruit have been used for years for weight loss, they were pure, real and applied to the skin as well as smelled. It wasn't until just the scent was singled out for use and chemically manufactured that things went askew. This book takes into consideration the confusion many have over how to use Aromatherapy for a true healing effect and the effects essences or Aromacology may have on the body as well. All healing recipes use pure essential oils, preferably steam distilled and organic. In the case of fragrance oils, they are used for what their name implies…fragrancing things and creating perfumes.

Another form of flower use which also gets frequently confused with Aromatherapy by lay people are flower essences which are at times teamed up with gem essences. A branch of Bach flower essences, flower and gem essences are decoction/infusions of botanicals or stones in alcohol. Unlike Aromatherapy or even Aromacology, very, very little is known about any beneficial effects of essences. People are not *healed* by flower essences because they have a specific health concern but instead because there is an underlying condition which is somehow addressed by the essence, (i.e. low self worth, frigidness, etc.). In a way, it's likened to the thinking of pre-fifth century B.C. that supernatural powers control ones wellness but slightly updated for a modern society's view about reality. Once again, as with Aromacology, Aromatherapy was used as a way of bringing recognition to essence use. Most people understood the basic concepts of Aromatherapy, but not essence use. Therefore the merging of the two served to bring more people into using essences but also did much to confuse about the real healing effects of Aromatherapy. Currently there is very little if any research showing that treating oneself with flower essences really serves any purpose at all except on a purely placebo basis. As mentioned above, gem essences are also created to be used in conjunction with the flower essences. Is it reasonable to think you can actually get an essence from a stone or mineral? The type of essence that people whom believe in flower essence use are referring to is the inherent "nature, spirit or quality" of the object. So, the actual essence in the perfume context is not what is being extracted but instead the spirit of the flower or stone. A popular belief of Dark Age alchemists, essence use hasn't really become as popular as other forms of traditional healing and with good reason. Just as with Aromacology, the body as a whole isn't being taken into consideration. When you cut yourself, it isn't because you are having low self-esteem, instead it is because you had an unforeseen accident. Your body, the cut area, needs immediate attention and so does your mind. You need something that will calm you down and lastly your mind to keep you optimistic about the days ahead even though you just had an accident. Essential oils and Aromatherapy have a very long tract record for addressing all of these aspects of the body and the same is true with herbology. When one starts attempting to peel away what they think is not needed, things begin to unravel and what once worked so well, fails to work at all. Self diagnosis is also very inherent to the use of essences and unless you have a degree in psychology, this can be very hard not to mention dangerous. Flower essence use seems best implemented for people under long term professional counseling by a psychologist but should not be used in the place of medications prescribed. Some attempt to make flower essences a cure all, which is pretty impossible due to the original thought about it's healing actions which many fail to fully understand. I have included a chapter on Bach Flower remedies because it has been in use longer and is more realistic about it's limitations. Dr. Bach also had a more professional view about how to use essences.

Law of Signatures & Herbology

Herbology is another ancient form of floral use. The petals, flower heads and other portions of the plant were dried or used fresh in a number of applications. The most common being in the form of decoctions/infusions, salves, poultices, creams, syrups, etc., and even as snuff power. But how did people know which flowers were used for what, especially when libraries and/or paper was non-existent. Oral history can go but so far and could die out with whole groups of people in catastrophic events. So comes in one of the oldest forms of medicinal plant identification…*Signatures*. Believed to have been first started in ancient Greece, manuscripts containing signature botanicals were circulated throughout the Middle East and Europe and was also the basis of physician teachings. Simply by looking at a plant and it's growing surroundings, people and physicians believed they could decipher the secret healing benefits inherent to them. Flowers were more favored because so much could be discerned from the flower head and petals. Color was especially helpful. Red denoted astringency of the botanical and most plants with red flowers were used for blood ailments, especially in the case of purifying the blood and associated organs. Yellow flowers denoted a botanical that would be beneficial to the liver and gallbladder. They were also used to teat urinary tract problems and to rid the body of impurities. Blue and purplish flowers were used for sleep and relaxing ones spirits. Proper rest was thought to speed up recovery after illness and such blue botanicals were added to blends to induce deep sleep. In addition to the color, other aspects of the plant was looked at including the leaf shape, formation of the stems, what condition they were growing in and even if they were growing next to running water. A plant growing next to running water was thought to have somewhat different healing properties than the exact same species growing atop a high mountain. Although ancient signatures would sometimes have highly different explanations for healing properties for the above reason, they may have been on to something, in the area of standardization. Plants growing in mineral rich soil may have a slightly different level of healing qualities as opposed to plants growing in depleted soil. On the other hand, plants growing in the same soil conditions have been found to have differing healing properties as well. This can be due to a number of reason including sun and atmospheric conditions.

Signatures have become the basis of many ancient forms of healing now popular today including classical Western herbalism and Unani Tibb, the herbal healing of the Arabs and later South Asians. Many of the signatures, first collected and recorded in one place by Theophrastus back in 3 B.C. are still considered useful in modern herbology. Unlike thinking prior to signatures, that illness was caused by supernatural powers, herbs were prescribed to put ones health back in balance and as preventative medicine in the case of plagues and widespread disease.

Flowers for Healing

When you prepare your own remedies and concoctions, it is always important to use the best ingredients you can! This means, in the case of Aromatherapy, to use pure, steam distilled essential oils that are of a professional or Aromatherapy grade. Being organically grown/wild crafted is always a major plus. Using cheap, inferior essential oils will end up giving you not only dismal results but also the chance of severe skin reactions. Many $5.00 essential oils are no more than misrepresented fragrance oils and hold no real healing benefit at all, except perhaps on an Aromacology plane. This will not help you if you are attempting to clear your skin of acne or give highlights to your hair. Be very mindful of the essential oil you are buying and it's quality. In the back of this book there is a list of companies that provide mail-order supply of high quality essential oils, if you are leery of the selection in your local health food/drug store, use them. Being that essential oils are very concentrated, one small bottle will last you a long time if you store them properly.

Flowers in the form of dried and fresh also need to be careful picked. The best way of being assured you are using the highest quality floral botanicals is to grow them yourself. Even if all you have is a window box or patio planter, growing your own medicinal flowers is not only rewarding but also perfect for culinary uses. Growing and drying your own flowers is not as hard as you think, especially if you grow flowers indicated for your zone or climate. Further information is given later on in this book and in the notes area in the form of great and very helpful websites! Culinary wise, you must be extremely careful about where you obtain your flowers. It can not be stressed more to never use flowers from a florist or that has been gathered into a bouquet as these flowers have been heavily treated with chemicals that should not be ingested. At times, these flowers are also dyed and most likely were heavily sprayed with pesticides when they were growing. Genetic altering is yet another concern as is radiation which is at times used on plants. I recommend growing your own flowers for culinary use as you can be assured they are completely organic. Few flowers are grown commercially for consumption so your health is not taken into consideration in the growing process. The same can be said for flowers used for healing unless the farmer knows they will be turned into tea or something of the like. It isn't worth taking the risk, grow your own flowers and cultivate them as you see fit. This can include giving them only filtered water and organic soil or sprinkling a few seeds in front of your house.

· Chapter One ·
The Flowers

Therapeutic Index

Aches & Soreness:
Chamomile (Roman & German works), Lavender, Comfrey, Rosemary
Acne:
Chamomile (Roman & German both work well), Geranium*, Violet, Lavender*, Dandelion, Soapwort
Allergies:
Chimomile (Roman & German both work well), Lavender*
Artritis:
Horseradish, Chamomile*, Thyme*, Sage, Rosemary, Comfrey, Feverfew
Athelete's Foot:
Lavender, Marigold, Red Clover
Boils & Blisters:
Chamomile (German & Roman works)*, Lavender, Echinacea (Purple Coneflower), Golden rod, Golden seal, St. John's Wort, Geranium*, Comfrey
Bronchitis:
Lavender, White Horehound, Violet, Golden seal, Thyme, Coltsfoot, Mullein
Bruises:
Arnica*, Geranium, Lavender, Comfry, St. John's Wort, Violet, Calendula, Borage, Bugle, Hyssop
Burnes:
Chamomile (German & Roman works)*, Geranium, Lavender, Marigold, Marshmallow
Childbirth Aids:
Jasmine, Lavender, Rose*

Cuts & Sores:
Chamomile (Roman & German works), Geranium, Lavender, Marigold, Dandelion, Golden seal, Yarrow, Hyssop, Comfrey

Depression:
Jasmine, Rose, Lavender, Orange blossom*, Chamomile, Geranium, Thyme

Eczema:
Chamomile (Roam & German works), Geranium, Lavender, Marigold, Fumitory, Rose, Violet, Red Clover, Yarrow (Milfoil) , Marshmallow

Greasy & Overly Oily Skin:
Geranium, Jasmine, Lavender, Marigold, Elder flower, Rose

Hair Care:
Arnica*, Rosemary, Chamomile (Roman), Yarrow, Soapwort

Headaches:
Lavender, Chamomile (Roman & German works), Rose, Rose hips, Skullcap, Violet, Feverfew, Linden, Lily of the Vally, Primrose, Thyme

Indigestion:
Chamomile (Roman or German works), Lavender, Yarrow, Thyme, Violet

Insect Bites:
Chamomile (German & Roman works), Lavender*, Marigold, Bee Balm, Thyme

Insect Repellents:
Geranium, Lavender, Red Clover, Feverfew

Insomia:
Chamomile (German & Roman works), Lavender, Orange blossom*, Rose, Violet, Yarrow, Neroli, Marshmallow, Bee balm, Cowslip

Menopausal Problems:
Geranium, Jasmine, Rose, Evening primrose (oil)

Palpitations:
Orange blossom*, Rose*

PMS:
Chamomile (Roman & German works), Geranium*, Lavender, Orange blossom, Bee balm

Poor Circulation:
Geranium, Orange blossom, Rose, Violet, Lavender*

Rashes:
Chamomile (German & Roman works), Lavender, Marigold

Rheumatism:
Chamomile (Roman & German works), Lavender, Violet

Scares & Stretch Markes:

Lavender, Orange blossom*, Violet
Vertigo:
Lavender, Violet
Weight Loss:
Rosemary, Geranium*, Lavender
Wrinkles & Aging Skin:
Geranium, Jasmine, Lavender, Orange blossom*, Rose*, Cowslip
* means essential oils of this plant works best

In-dpeth Look Into Medicinal Flowers

Here you will find a comprehensive alphabetical list of many flowers you probably already know about but never thought to use medicinally. In this all told section you will learn everything you need to know to safely use the healing power of flowers to your advantage, both preventatively and for treatment of self-limiting ailments. Learn the traditional thought behind their medicinal usage along with modern day findings.

Rose

"...the decoction of red Roses made with wine and used, is very good for the headache, and pains in the eyes, ears, throat, and gums; as also for the fundament, the lower part of the belly and the matrix, being bathed or put into them..."-Nicholas Culpeper, 1653

Common name: Rose
Latin name: *Rosa spp.*
Also known as: by many local and spp. names
Origins: China
Parts used: Flowers, leaves, fruit (rose hips)
Healing actions: The rose has many uses including aromatic and culinary. The petals have been longed use to produce expensive essential oil which contains antiseptic, antiviral, antidepressant, sedative, laxative, and hemostatic qualities and is used for rejuvenating the skin. Rose water extracts were used for flavoring confections and petals and hips were turned into jams, jellies, tea, syrups and wine. Externally, rose is very healing to the skin and can be used to help heal scars and reduce age lines.

Greater Periwinkle

"...vehemently tormented with the cramp for a long while which could be by no means eased till he had wrapped some of the branches [of periwinkle] hereof about his limbs..."-Williams Coles, 1657

Common name: Periwinkle
Latin name: *Vinca major*
Also known as: Sorcerer's violet

Oragins: Europe

Parts used: Flowers, laves

Healing actions: The leaves have been used to lesson menstrual bleeding and as a tonic to reduce blood pressure. An infusion has been made traditionally to clean small wounds as it has astringent qualities.

Yucca

Common name: Yucca

Latin name: *Yucca filamentosa*

Also known as: Needle palm

Origins: United States

Parts used: Flowers, leaves, fruit, roots

Healing actions: An important plant to the Native American Indians such as the Hopi of the South West United States, it has many traditional uses especially culinary wise. The flowers, fruit and stalks were eaten as daily fare. Externally it was turned into a salve to treat skin conditions such as sores and internally taken as a tea to treat old age problems like arthritis. Yucca was also used for cleaning the hair and body as it has astringent and soap like qualities.

Marsh Mallow

"…the juice of Mallows boiled in old oil and applied, takes away all roughness of the skin, as also the scurf, dandriff, or dry scabs on the head, or other parts, if they be anointed therewith, or washed with the decoction, and preserves the hair from falling off…"-Nicholas Culpeper, 1653

Common name: Marsh Mallow

Latin name: *Althaea officinalis*

Also known as: Hock herb, Mallards, Cheeses, Althea

Origins: Europe

Parts used: Flowers, leaves, seeds, roots

Healing actions: Frequently used in culanry raw dishes, marsh mallow which has been used since Egyptian times has traditionally been turned into a tea or tonic to treat gastric disorders including ulcers and diarrhea. A poiltice was also made to healp healin skin conditions.

Lavender

"…a decoction made with the flowers of Lavender, Hore-hound, Fennel and Asparagus root, and a little Cinnamon, is very profitably used to help the falling-sickness, and the giddiness or turning of the brain: to gargle the mouth with the decoction thereof is good against the tooth-ache…" -Nicholas Culpeper, 1653

Common name: Lavender

Latin name: *Lavandula spp.*

Also known as: by many local and spp. names
Origins: Mediterranean
Parts used: Flowers, leaves
Healing actions: There are over 28 species of the wonderful plant which has many healing and culinary uses. Tea prepared from the flowers have been traditionally used for headaches, dizziness, nausea and anxiety problems. It has also been used to lower high blood pressure and aid in menstrual problems. Externally, compresses of flower waters or hydrosuls and essential oils can be used to treat chronic skin conditions such as acne and aid in the healing process of minor burns. It's been long revered as a beauty treatment as well and was used to scent bedding which in turn helped one fall asleep faster and repel insects. Lavender contains antidepressant, antiseptic, analgesic, antispasmodic, nervine, sedative, and hypotensive qualities.

Safty note: Should not be used in high amounts during pregnancy as it is a uterine stimulant.

Arnica

Common name: Arnica
Latin name: *Arnica montana*
Also known as: Leopard's bane
Origins: Europe and Asia
Parts used: Flowers, leaves, roots
Healing actions: Used externally to treat chronic skin conditions and to help heal bruses, muscle pain and sprains. Due to it's toxic nature when ingested, external and homeopathic use is only recommended and caution should be taken not to allow it access to open wounds or broken skin.

Lawn Daisy

"…an ointment made thereof doth wonderfully help all wounds that have inflammations about them, or by reason of moist humours having access unto them, are kept long from healing, and such are those, for the most part, that happen to joints of the arms or legs…"-Nicholas Culpeper, 1653

Common name: Daisy
Latin name: *Bellis perennis*
Also known as: English daisy
Origins: Europe and Asia
Parts used: Flowers, leaves
Healing actions: Used in faw culanry dishes, the flowers have been traditionally used in infusions for skin washes and bath addatives to treat the body and skin of eczema, dry skin, acne and other conditions. The flowers can also be turned into a tonic tea.

Safty note: The daisy can provoke excisting allergies.

Perennial Chamomile

"…the bathing with a decoction of Camomile takes away weariness, eases pains, to what part of the body soever they be applied…"-Nicholas Culpeper, 1653

Common name: Roman Chamomile

Latin name: *Chamamelum nobile*

Also known as: English chamomile, Sweet chamomile, True chamomile, Camomile, Garden chamomile

Oragins: Europe

Parts used: Flowers, leaves

Healing actions: Chamomile is a very versatile botanical, traditionally used internationally, in the form of a tea, to treat digestive problems and aid in quality sleep. It has also been used to prevent nausea and urinary tract infections. Externally, chamomile can be used to aid the skin in healing and becoming more supple. The essential oil form of Roman chamomile has been used to help eating disorders such as anorexia and mental stress problems. It has been shown to contain antiseptic, analgesic, antiphlogistic, bactericidal and nerve sedative qualities.

Safty note: Some people with very sensative skin may find chamomile causes contact dermatitis.

Clove Pink

Common name: Pink

Latin name: *Dianthus caryophyllus*

Also known as: Gillyflower

Origins: Mediterranean

Parts used: Flowers

Healing actions: Used in many culinary applications including wines and soups, pinks were traditionally made into tea to give one more energy. It is mainly used for scenting poducts including soaps and perfumes.

Heliotrope

Common name: Heliotrope

Latin name: *Heliotropium arborescens*

Also known as: Cherry pie, Turnsole

Origins: Peru

Parts used: flower, leaf

Healing actions: Mainly used in the perfume industry to scent commercial products such as soap, it was traditionally used by the Inca indians to treat feverish conditions.

Echinacea

Common name: Echinacea
Latin name: *Echinacea angustifolia*
Also knows as: Purple cone flower, Black sampson
Origins: United States
Parts used: Roots
Healing actions: Echinacea has been found to aid the immune system in defending the body from colds and flu and may even reduce allergy problems. Frequently used in tea form, it has antiviral and immune stimulating qualities.

Safety note: High doses can cause dizziness and nausea.

Hyssop
"...it helps to expectorate tough phlegm, and is effectual in all cold griefs or diseases of the chests or lungs, being taken either in syrup or licking medicine..."-Nicholas Culpeper, 1653

Common name: Hyssop
Latin name: *Hyssopus officinalis*
Also known as: Issopo celestino
Origins: Europe
Parts used: Flowers, leaves
Healing actions: Traditionally used in the digestion of fatty food, an infusion may be made to act as a mild sedative and to bring up phlegm from the flu, colds and bronchitis. Externally, the leaves may be used in a poultice or plaster to help heal wounds and bruises.

Safety note: High doses of the essential oil form can induce convultions.

St. John's Wort
"...it is a singular wound herb; boiled in wine and drank, it heals inward hurts or bruises; made into an ointment, it open obstructions, dissolves swellings, and closes up the lips of wounds..."-Nicholas Culpeper, 1653

Common name: St. John's Wort
Latin name: *Hypericum perforatum*
Also known as: Hypericum
Origins: Europe and China
Parts used: Flowers, leaves, fruit
Healing actions: It has many external applications including use on minor burns, swelling, vericose veins, hemorrhoids and wounds and was used to treat poor blood circulation. Internally it was used to treat poor sleep and diarrhea. In 1977 it was declared unsafe by the US Food & Drug Administration as cows given high amounts of it to eat became very sensetive to sun and blistered. This decleration was partially reversed, allowing it to be sold in tincture form only. Today it is used to treat minor depression and mood swings.

Safety note: May cause contact dermatitis. Should not be taken at the same time as other prescription antidepressant drugs or MAO-inhibitors. Food interactions may also occur when combined with yogurt, chococlate, or pickled items and one should never cunsume beer, wine or coffee while using St. John's Wort. People who are fair skined should also obstain from it's constant use.

Madonna Lily
Common name: Madonna Lily
Latin name: *Lilium candidum*
Also known as: Bourbon lily
Oragins: Mediterranen
Parts used: Flower, roots
Healing actions: The roots were used to create an ointment to treat chronic skin conditions such as acne and problems like burns, boils and insect bites. The petals of the flower can also be used to create an infused oil to treat eczema.

Musk Mallow
Common name: Musk Mallow
Latin name: *Malva moschata*
Also known as: Cuteleaf mallow
Origins: Europe and Africa
Parts used: Flowers, leaves, roots
Healing actions: Not to be confused with marsh mallow, the flowers and young shoots contain many vitamins including B, A and C. It has also been turned into caugh syrups and skin preperations to conditions and soothe.

Begamot
Common name: Bergamot
Latin name: *Mondarda didyma*
Also known as: Bee balm, Scarlet monarda
Origins: United States
Parts used: Flowers, leaves
Healing actions: The Native American Indians brewed bergamot and called it Oswego tea which aided in the releaf of cold symptoms. The flowers were also infused in oil to produce hair and skin treatments.

Primrose
Common name: Primrose
Latin name: *Primula vulgaris*
Also known as: Spring primula
Origins: Europe
Parts used: Flowers, roots, leaves

Healing actions: Traditionally used in love potions, primrose can be used in culinary dishes and in tea to help one sleep better and to relieve headaches. A infusion or decoction of the plant can be used for many external applications including for the treatment of acen and for clensing the body.

Safty note: May cause contact dematitis. Do not use if you have an allergy to asprin or pregnant as it is a utarin stimulant. People taking blood thinning prescription drugs should also avoid use of primrose.

Gardenia

Common name: Gardenia
Latin name: *Gardenia jasminoides*
Also known as: Zhi-zi, Cape jasmine, Gardinia, Common gardenia
Origins: China and Jasmine
Parts used: Flowers, leaves, fruit, root
Healing actions: In traditional Chinese medicine the roots are used to detoxify the system and clear up feverish conditions such as the flu. The essential oil is mainly used in the perfume industry and has not been found to hold noticeable healing abilities.

Sacred Lotus

Common name: Lotus Flower
Latin name: *Nelumbo nucifera*
Also known as: Lotus lily
Origins: Asia and Australia
Parts used: Flowers, leaves, seeds, roots
Healing actions: The rhizome of the flower is turned into a juice which is said to help heal acne, eczema and other chronic skin conditions. The seeds have been used to treat heart conditions and reduce feverish conditions. The stamens of the flowers can be turned into an aromatic tea which may help the heart.

Soap Wort

Common name: Soapwort
Latin name: *Saponaria officinalis*
Also known as: Bouncing bet
Origins: Asia and Europe
Parts used: Flowers, leaves, roots
Healing actions: The leaves of soapwort contain saponins which soften water and clense like soap and have been used to wash hair, skin and clothing. It can also be used to treat chronic skin conditions such as acne and psoriasis.

Safty note: The plant can be toxic when taken internally.

Dandelion

"…it is of an opening and cleansing quality, and therefore very effectual for the obstructions of the liver, gall and spleen, and the diseases that arise from them…"-Nicholas Culpeper, 1653

Common name: Dandelion
Latin name: *Taraxacum set. Ruderalia spp.*
Also known as: Fairy clock, Lion's tooth, Wild endive
Origins: Northen Hemisphere
Parts used: Flowers, leaves, seeds, roots

Healing actions: A strong diuretic and liver clenser, dandelion is rich in both vitamins C and A. It also has been traditionally used to clear acne and other minor skin conditions externally and internally. Dandlion has also been found to prevent and control yeast infections, high blood presure and as a digestive aid.

Borage

"…the leaves and roots are to very good purpose used in putrid and pestilential fevers, to defend the heart, and help to resist and expel the poison, or the venom of other creatures…"-Nicholas Culpeper, 1953

Common name: Borage
Latin name: *Borago officinalis*
Also known as: Star flower
Origins: Europe
Parts used: Flowers, seeds, leaves

Healing actions: A tea can be made with the flowers to releave fevers, help caughs, depression and stress. Borage has also been traditionally used to promote milk flow in nursing mothers and in natural caugh syrups.

Calendula

"…it hath pleasant, bright and shining yellow flowers, the which do close at the setting downe of the sunne, and do spread and open againe at the sunne rising…"-Dodoens-Lyte, 1578

Common name: Calendula
Latin name: *Calendula officinalis*
Also known as: Pot marigold
Origins: Europe and Mediterranean
Parts used: Flowers, leaves

Healing actions: An infusion can be made of the flowers and used to simulate the liver and for releaving stomache pains. It can also be turned into a cream or infused oil to treat chronic skin conditions and inflammations such as acne, eczema, dry skin, minor wounds, burns and sore nipples.

Feverfew

"…the decoction thereof made with some sugar, or honey put thereto, is used by many with good success to help the cough and stuffing of the chest, by colds, as also to cleanse the reins and bladder, and help to expel the stone in them…"- Nicholas Culpeper, 1653

Common name: Feverfew
Latin name: *Tanacetum parthenium*
Also known as: Featherfoil, Wild quinie, Beachelor's button, Febrifuge plant
Origins: Europe
Parts used: Flowers, leaves

Healing actions: Feverfew tea was traditionally used to treat irregular menstrual periods and after childbirth. The flowers, when infused in oil, have been used to treat migraine headaches and reduce arthritic swelling at the joints.

Safety note: Chewing the fresh leaves may cause irritation and inflammation of the mouth including ulcers. People taking blood thinning prescription drugs should also avoid it's use completly as with pregnent women.

Queen Anne's Lace

Common name: Queen Anne's Lace
Latin name: *Daucus carota*
Also known as: Wild carrot
Origins: India and Europe
Parts used: Flowers, roots seeds

Healing actions: The roots of queen anne's lace are rich in vitamin C and have long been used as a berverage and source for natural dye. A tea can be created and used to substate cooffee yet act as a diuretic as coffee does. It also has bacterialcidal qualities and may lower blood presure if consumed regularly.

Red Clover

Common name: Clover
Latin name: *Trifolium pratense*
Also known as: Meadow trefoil, Sweet clover, Cow clower, Purple clover
Origins: Europe
Parts used: Flower, roots, leaves, seeds

Healing actions: The flowers can be turned into a sweet tea as well as a skin cream to treat minor skin problems, such as dryness. Many believe clover flowers contain anti-cancer agents which is being further reasearched. In high amounts, clover has been found to act as a natural estrogen replacement to women.

Safty note: People with a history of strokes or bloodclotting problems should avoid clover. Women taking birth control pills should also be careful.

Sunflower

Common name: Sunflowers
Latin name: *Helianthus annuus*
Also known as: Chimalati
Origins: United States
Parts used: Flowers, leaves, seeds, roots
Healing actions: The roots have a laxative quality and may be turned into a tonic for that application. They also aid in relieving stomach pain. The seeds can be used to treat coughs and as a diuretic.

Forget Me Not
Common name: Forget-Me-Not
Latin name: *Myosotis sylvatica*
Also known as: Mouse Ears
Origins: Europe, Asia and Africa
Parts used: Flower, leaves
Healing actions: Used in culinary dishes and homeopathic remadies, it can be used externally to treat wounds and heal minor skin conditions.

Honeysuckle
Common name: Honeysuckle
Latin name: *Lonicera japonica*
Also known as: Gold or Silver flower
Origins: Asia
Parts used: Flowers
Healing actions: Teas can be made from the flowers and used to lower blood sugar levels, detoxify the system and to treat colds and flu. Externally, a tonic can be made to help heal minor skin conditions and for swollen lymph glands.

Safety note: Any berries that form on the honeysuckle should not be ingested in any way as they are poisonous.

Nasturtium
Common name: Nasturtium
Latin name: *Tropaeolum majus*
Also known as: Indian Cress
Origins: South America
Parts used: Flowers, fruit, leaves, seeds
Healing actions: The seeds of nasturium can be used in an infusion to treat colds and coughs. The whole plant can be used as a tonic for the hair and scalp and was traditionally thought of as a aphrodisiac.

Mullein

"…a decoction of the leaves hereof, and of Sage, Marjoram, and Camomile flowers, and the places bathed therewith, that have sinews stiff with cold or cramps, doth bring them much ease and comfort…"-Nicholas Culpeper, 1653

Common name: Mullein

Latin name: *Verbascum thapsus*

Also known as: Toches, Verbascum, Candlewick, Velvet dock, Aaron's rod, Lungwort, Flannel plant, Shepheard's staff

Origins: Flowers, leaves, roots

Healing actions: Native American Indians used mullein as an incense that was burned to reawaken those who unconscious. It was also smoked with other herbs and tabacco. The flowers can be used to help heal chronic skin conditions and the oil produced from the seeds can soothe the skin. The root can be turned into a tonic and used as a diuretic. It has been shown to releave hemorrhoids when applied.

Safty note: The seeds of the mullein are extremly toxic and can poison if ingested.

Angelica

"…a water distilled from the root simply, as steeped in wine, and distilled in a glass, is much more effectual than the water of the leaves; and this water, drank two or three spoonfuls at a time, easeth all pains and torments coming of cold…" -Nicholas Culpeper, 1653

Common name: Angelica

Latin name: *Angelica spp.*

Also known as: Dang gui, Wild celery, Masterwort

Origins: Europe and Asia

Parts used: Leaves, roots

Healing actions: The main uses for angelica include that of digestive and bronchial problems. An infusion can be made of either the roots or leaves to help treat these two conditions. A cream and massage oil can also be made to treat minor skin irritations and arthritic problems.

Safaty note: Do not use if prenant as it is a strong utarin stimulant. Diabetics should not use either as it contains a high sugar content. Never use the fresh root as it's poisonous.

Wild Passion Flower

Common name: Passion Flower

Latin name: *Passiflora incarnata*

Also known as: Maypop, Water lemon, Apricot vine

Origins: United States

Parts used: Flowers, fruit, laves, roots

Healing actions: Native American Indians used passion flower as a full body tonic and for irritated eyes. It can also be used to treat minor burns and skin irritations. The leaves can be used as a tea ro help lower blood pressure and lesson insomnia. Passionflower was long used as an additive to sleep inducing medications until 1978 when the Food & Drug Administration banned it from such products due to lack of medicals findings at that time. Today, passionflower has been found to indeed containe complex traquilizer and sedative qualities which are being further looked into. While sedative, it is nonnarcotic so there is no pissiblity of habit forming side-effects.

Safty note: Passionflower has been found to be a uterine stimulant and should be avoided by pregnent women.

Yarrow

Common name: Yarrow

Latin name: *Achillea millefolium*

Also known as: Nosebleed, Thousand weed, Soldier's woundworth, Bloodwort, Milfoil

Origins: Europe

Parts used: Flowers, leaves

Healing actions: Traditionally it was used to help stop bleeding and heal wounds. A tea infusion may be made and used to treat colds, the flu and poor circulation problems. It can also be used to treat hay fever and other allergies. Due to it's containing small amounts of a substance called thujone, it can be used as a mild sedative or tranquilizer.

Safety note: Should not be used by prenant women as it's a utarin stimulant or by people with very sensative skin or allergies to ragweed as rashes may develope.

Violets

"…all the Violets are cold and moist while they are fresh and green, and are used to cool any heat, or distemperature of the body, either inwardly or outwardly…"-Nicholas Culpeper, 1653

Common name: Violet

Latin name: *Viola odorata*

Also known as: Blue and Purple Violet, English Violet

Origins: Europe and Asia

Parts used: Leaves, flower and root

Healing actions: The leaves and flowers work wonders on various chronic skin conditions such as acne, eczema, etc. This is due to its anti-inflammatory qualities. Violet also works to improve circulation and certain pulmonary conditions. There are over 200 species which grow world wide today with Parma and Victoria being most popular in use by perfumers. Primarily used today in the food industry as flavoring for confections.

Safety note: Avoid in high amounts as nausea may occur.

· Chapter Two ·

Aromatherapy

Aromatherapy is the use of pure essential oils, many of which are extracted from flowers, for health and healing. They are applied topically and used aromatically for a great number of ailments. Essential oils are derived from many pounds of plant matter, producing a highly concentrated oil like substance. These oils contain all of the medicinal properties along with the vitamins and nutrients the plant has to offer. Although scientists try, they are only barely able to replicate the scent of many flowers and never the pure essential oils which are extracted from their leaves, petals, roots, etc. This is why it is always important to use pure essential oils and never fragrance oils for Aromatherapy.

The art of Aromatherapy has a rich and long history, believed to have originated with and mastered by the ancient Egyptians, most notably for the practice of embalming. Oils derived from cedarwood and myrrh along with other sacred aromatics were used for the mummification's. Various skin and hair preparations, for the living, were also prepared with the use of essential oils. The art of using aromatic oils for beauty, perfumery and health spread across Asia and Europe with the coming of better trade routes. The Greeks used essential oils for all sorts of perfumes and healing remedies. Romans took it one step further by perfuming everything, including clothing, bedding, homes, hair and body. In the time of plagues and other sicknesses which swept many parts of Europe, essential oil use became a way of surviving. Women's gloves, in the 18th century were scented with special perfume concoctions and sold to women, handkerchiefs were also soaked with oils to be placed over the face while walking the streets because of the awful odor and soot in the air. Many inventions were made as a form of defense which utilized essential oils, especially lavender, disinfecting qualities. People are rediscovering how important essential oils are and how they can be used for healing as well as preventative measures.

Essential oil extraction methods

One of the most important things to remember is that if you want the best outcome from using a certain essential oil, be sure to find the best quality Aromatherapy grade oil. Beware of so called essential oil product lines that offer all their oils for the same low price. Flowers such as the rose do not yield the same amount of essential oil as other botanicals so it is always more expensive, if it is pure and real. Some essential oils are pre-mixed in a base oil of almond, etc. While this is fine and even preferable for use on the skin and hair, they are not as effective when used for scenting purposes and for inhalation. One can always dilute a pure essential oil, so if you want to use your same essential oil for many projects and application, look for ones that are not pre-diluted. Certain oils, such as Lemongrass is often used to contaminate other essential oils and create a filler effect. Always read the label carefully, to make sure the essential oil you are buying is pure. If there isn't a label, pass on buying that particular brand. Although hard to find at times, essential oils derived from organically grown or wildcrafted plants are always preferable. When a plant is sprayed with chemicals and then turned into an essential oil, the pesticides are also included in a concentrated form. When you use these oils, the impurities can end up in your blood steam doing more harm than good. Lastly, try to obtain oils that are steamed distilled. Steam distillation involves the plant being placed in a still like contraption which forces hot steam through the plant material. The steam is trapped in piping which is cold and condenses the steam back into a liquid state. Floating at the top of the collected water, the essential oils can be found. The oil is skimmed off and bottled and the rest is turned into floral waters which are used in soaps and other products. Unfortunately, many companies have turned to the chemical solvent method of extraction. Just as with the pesticide problem, the companies are never able to remove all of the solvent and some is left in the finished product. This may be a cheaper way of doing things but the end product is not of the same quality.

Many people mistakenly think essential oils are like perfumes or fragrances which can be applied directly to the skin. Unless it is mixed fist in a carrier oil of almond, vegetable, olive, etc., never apply right to the skin. Many essential oils are concentrated enough to take varnish and finishes off of furniture so think of what they can do to your skin. They are highly concentrated and need to be handled accordingly. Even after being mixed in a carrier oil or diluted in water, some essential oils may prove irritating. Citrus oils such as orange and mint oils fall into this category and should be used with caution by people with sensitive skin.. Most oils derived from flowers are not as irritating. It is always important to do a patch test first to make sure you will not develop a rash or allergic reaction from the product containing essential oils, especially when you make it yourself.

Aromatherapy essential oil blending chart

When essential oils are combined with certain other oils, they can form a synergistic blend that is more potent and effective on a particular application. Use the chart below to find which oils enhance each other in a healing synergistic manor. We will stick to oils derived from flowering plants and trees.

Chamomile (Roman)......Lavender, Rose, Geranium, Neroli, Melissa, Lemon, Ylang Ylang

Chamomile (German) ....Rose, Geranium, Lavender, Jasmine, Marjoram

Geranium ....Bergamot, Lavender, Lemon grass, Rose

Gardenia ....Rose, Jasmine, Tuberose, Neroli

Labdanum......................Chamomile, Lavender, Bergamot

Jasmine ....Neroli, Rose, Cedarwood, Clary sage

Marigold ....Mandarin orange

Violet ....Hyacinth, Tuberose

Lavender ....Geranium, Bergamot, Chamomile, Rosemary, Pine

Neroli ....Rose, Jasmine, Lavender, Bergamot, Myrrh

Rose ....Jasmine, Geranium, Neroli

Narcissus ....Jasmine, Neroli

Cassie ....Bergamot, Violet, Ylang Ylang

Rosemary.......................Bergamot, Cedarwood, Lavender, Thyme

Thyme............................Rosemary, Orange, Lemon, Bergamot

Boronia ....Bergamot, Violet, Clary sage

Hyacinth ....Violet, Jasmine, Neroli, Ylang Ylang

Tuberose ....Gardenia, Jasmine, Violet, Neroli, Ylang Ylang

Medicinal Aromatherapy Chart

In this chart you will find the medicinal qualities of essential Aromatherapy oils which are derived from flowers. If you wish to use an essential oils remember to use only Aromatherapy grade essential oils and not a fragrance oil. Try to find oils that come from organically grown plants and that are steam distilled. Otherwise you may have an essential oil product contaminated with large amounts of toxic pesticides and other chemicals.

Chamomile (Roman)......Anti-inflammatory, Antiseptic, Bactericidal, Insomnia, Calming nerves, Sprains, Nerve sedative, Hair-care, Anti-depressant, Chronic skin conditions

Chamomile (German) ....Anti-inflammatory, Bactericidal, Antispasmodic, nervous system sedative, Tension headaches

Geranium ....Astringent, Anti-inflammatory, Astringent, Antiseptic, Antidepressant, Promotes dermal healing, Diuretic, Deodorant, relieves menstrual problems

Geranium (Rose) ....Antidepressant, Nerve sedative, Memory enhancer

Gardenia ....Antiseptic qualities, Aphrodisiac

Labdanum......................Antiseptic, Astringent, Antimicrobial, Skin care

Jasmine ....Antidepressant, Antiseptic, Aphrodisiac, Anti-inflammatory, Sedative, Menstrual pain, Cramps, respiratory problems

Calamintha ....Antiseptic, Astringent, Sedative, Cramps

Marigold ....Anti-inflammatory, Astringent, Fungicide, Antiseptic, Antispasmodic, Dry skin conditions, Vericose Veins

Violet ....Anti-inflammatory, Diuretic, Stimulant, Acne, chronic skin conditions

Lavende........................Analgesic, Antibiotic, Antimicrobial, Anti-inflammatory, Headaches, Acne, Diuretic, Sedative, Stimulant, Deodorant, Insect bites

Exotic Verbena...............Antiseptic, Sedative, Deodorant, Chills, Headaches, Muscle pain

Neroli ....Antidepressant, Sedative, works on cases of shock, Antispasmodic, Aphrodisiac, Fungicidal, mild Stimulant, Anxiety reliever, Hemorrhoids, Hypnotic

Rose ....Antidepressant, Antiviral, Astringent, Bactericidal, Stimulating, Aging skin, Acne, Circulation, Sedative

Cassie ....Aphrodisiac, Antiseptic, Insecticide

Arnica ....Anti-inflammatory, Stimulant, Burns

What to Use as a Carrier Oil

Essential oils should always be blended in a carrier oil before being applied to the skin. They also help to keep your essential oil from evaporating. Essential oils are quite volatile and will dissipate as soon as they are released from their glass bottle, which should be cobalt blue or deep brown. There are many oils to choose from, each with their own healing qualities. Try to find ones that will work with and to improve your skin type. The ones below have little or no scent of their own so they will not cover up the fragrance of the added essential oil.

Almond Oil

This great, scentless oil is wonderful for blending for use in beauty and massage treatments. Very easily found in most health food stores, it is highly nourishing to the skin and helps smooth and replenish it. Keep in mind that this oil needs to be kept in a cool, dry place and that it can go rancid fast if not. If you find any hint of odor, discard as this indicates rancidity..

Vegetable Oil

Salad oil may be used but because of it's heavy consistency, it works best when not used on the skin but instead, in a bath oil or on the hair. Works nicely on the hair as well or in combination with other carrier oils.

Jojoba Oil

A wonderful, light oil, jojoba actually resembles the natural oils given off by the human body. It works well in combination with other oils or as the main carrier oil for natural essential oil perfumes. Great for use on chronic skin conditions such as acne. If you notice any hint of odor, it has gone rancid, so discard it at once.

Olive Oil

While it works great for hair care treatments and on conditions such as arthritis, it's olive oil scent may over power the essential oils that are added. It can be combined with other carrier oils to dilute the smell a bit.

Grapeseed Oil

Light and clear it is perfect for skin and scalp treatments. Works great as the base for essential oil perfumes.

Sesame Oil

Try to buy the light version of this oil which is found in many Asian culinary dishes. Due to the deep amber color and pungent scent, it might totally cover up any essential oils you add. Try using it for bath oils or for hair treatments.

Sunflower Oil

The oil of the sunflower is quite healing and contains good amounts of vitamin F. Unfortunately is doesn't keep well. Try storing it in the refrigerator to extend the shellfire.

These additives are quite healing when added in small quantities to your blends.

Vitamin E

You can find Vitamin E oil in most stores nowadays either in capsule form or in a full bottle. Traditionally thought to help heal chronic skin conditions such acne, eczema, etc., some recent *small* study found otherwise. After seeing the pictures of the results myself, the scars using vitamin E oil did look worse. If you have found it helpful in the past, by all means use it. Further studies most certainly need to be done before vitamin E is ruled out for good. It however helps to preserve your blend and keeps the essential oils from evaporating and gives the carrier oil a longer shelf life.

Avocado Oil
Great addition to massage blends that will be used on sore muscles or cellulite problems. Add in small amounts to blends, as it may make the consistency of your concoction thick and sticky over time.

Benzion
Usually sold along side essential oils, benzion is really a gum that gets quite thick when kept in the refrigerator. It works well as a natural preservative but it does have a scent of it's own that may change your whole blend.

Calendula Oil
Add to blends that will be used on sore, bruised, chapped but unbroken skin. Works well to help relieve pain and swelling. Also is useful for skin preparations and treatments.

Carrot Oil
You will find this light oil wonderful for use on the skin. It of course contains a lot of betacarotene which is helpful in reversing some of the effects of the elements on the skin. Great addition to facial treatment blends.

Neem
This oil is a traditional Ayurvedic Indian oil derived from the Neem botanical and has been long used to heal the skin, especially in the cases of acne, and treat a number of conditions both externally and internally. It does, however, have a strong scent and may effect some aromatic blends.

Honey
A little acts as a natural preservative to massage blends and perfumes using essential oils. Too much may make the blend too thick and sticky. Honey has many humectant qualities and therefore helps the skin to retain it's natural moisture.

Aloe Gel

I have found using either vitamin C gel or Aloe Vera gel to be wonderful for diluting and suspending the essential oils. It also provides a greaseless cream when mixed with the essential oils, perfect for acne and oily skin conditions. Aloe in itself is good for cooling the skin and aiding in the healing of minor burns, wounds, too much sun and even fungal infections. Makes a great bath gel too for eczema skin conditions.

Ways of Using Essential Oils for Healing

There are many ways of using essential oils and adding their healing effects to your lifestyle. You will be surprised how easy it is to incorporate them in your daily routine. Over time you will find yourself replacing more and more store bought products which naturally prepared health aids containing natural, pure essential oils.

Inhalation

Use a large bowl that is heat safe and add essential oils before adding boiling water. Add water and place your face over it. Stay a comfortable distance away and as the water cools, move your face closer and closer to the water. Cover your head and the bowl with a towel for added benefit. This is a great way of purifying the skin and also for respiratory problems such as colds, coughs, etc. Try not to do this more then twice a week as your skin may get dried out or take on a skin condition called Jungle Acne.

Perfumes

Use a single essential oil and a carrier oil to create a wonderful and unique scent. Your perfume will have the added bonus of being uplifting if you pick an essential oil like Rose or calming if you choose Lavender. A few drops of essential oil of your choice can also be placed on a clean handkerchief and stored in your purse or pocket. Smell it anytime you need a calming or uplifting aromatic experience.

Compress

You can moisten a washcloth in hot or cold water and add a few drops of essential oil. This can be a great way of administrating the essential oil for sore muscles, headaches, chronic skin conditions, etc. Up to 5 drops will work nicely.

Room Fresherners and Purification

There are many ways of using essential oils for room freshening including candles, potpourris, steam, incense, aromatic lamps, lamp rings (for placement over low watt light bulbs), clay pots, mists, etc. Put a few drops anywhere that doesn't have a finish that can be taken off by the essential oil; for freshening with the added benefit of disinfecting the area. Essential oils can also be placed in a pot of simmering water on the stove over very low heat to fill the house with scent.

Baths
Essential oils can be added directly to the bath under the running water. It's best to enter the bath as soon as possible before the volatile oils evaporate before you can benefit from them. This application works wonderfully on soreness, achy joints, as well as skin conditions such as acne and circulatory problems. Instead of immersing your whole body, you can treat specific areas such as your feet in a warm foot bath. Up to 10 drops of essential oil may be used for a therapeutic effect. You may also make a bath oil by combining an essential oil and carrier oil.

Household Cleaners
Oils that are particularly disinfectant may be placed in water and sprayed throughout the house on hard surfaces to help kill germs naturally. This will help the whole family to stay healthier in the long run. The addition of only a few drops can do wonders.

Massage Oils
The most popular way of using Aromatherapy oil, massage oils can be specifically prepared for soreness, joint pain, certain skin conditions, moisturizing, etc. or they can be made just for their pleasing aroma and calming qualities. Easily concocted, simply pour enough carrier oil into a clean, glass or ceramic container and add the essential oils of your choice. 10 to 15 will do. About 5 drops of your massage oil will work nicely.

Hair Care
The great thing about essential oils is that they can be quickly added to almost anything, including commercially made products. If you can't live without your favorite store or salon bought shampoo or conditioner, you can enhance it with the power of Aromatherapy. Simply add 15 to 20 drops essential oil of choice to the entire container of product and shake well before using. Not only will it give you a pleasing scent but it will leave your hair better conditioned and shiny.

Make sure to keep the cap on tight and store in a cool, dry, place away from direct sunlight.

Skin Care

Just as with shampoos and conditioners, essential oils in smaller amounts can be added to your favorite moisturizer, toner, etc. Some companies are now making scent and color free versions of their line. This is preferable if you want to add essential oils for their scent and healing qualities. 5 to 10 drops will do, depending on the amount of product.

To help prolong the shelf life of your essential oils and make sure they retain their true medicinal qualities make sure to 1.) Keep them away from sunlight. Most essential oils come in a cobalt blue or deep brown bottle to help but it's best to store them in a tin or another container as well for added protection. Not doing so may lead to depletion of healing properties and total evaporation of the oil. 2.) Store in a cool, dry place to avoid evaporation of oil from high temperatures. You may also wish to store it in the refrigerator.

Some Therapeutic Blends

Remember to add your essential oil blend to a carrier oil such as vegetable or sweet almond before using it on your skin. Not doing so can lead to irritation and/or a rash. Also do a patch test before using all over the face or body. These same blends may be used in a sauna setting or bath as well instead of just massaging it in. If you do not have your own sauna, you can take a large, heat safe bowl or bucket and fill it with boiling water. Make sure to place it far away from where you will be sitting or standing in the shower. Add some essential oils of your choice and enjoy for 30 minutes or until water grows cold and stops producing steam. This works wonderfully for congestive and minor skin conditions.

Eczema:
10 drops Calendula, 10 Chamomile, 5 Geranium and 5 Lavender
Acne:
10 drops Chamomile, 10 drops Yarrow and 1 or 2 drops of Lavender
or
10 drops Rose, 10 Chamomile and 1 or 2 drops Lavender (optional)
Cellulite:
10 drops Rosemary and 8 Orange or Lemon
Sagging Skin:
15 drops Lavender, 5 drops Neroli and 10 drops Rose (optional)
Menstrual Pain:

10 drops Chamomile, 5 Jasmine and 5 drops Clary Sage
PMS:
10 drops Bergamot and 10 drops Rose
Colds:
10 drops Lavender and 10 drops Eucalyptus
Bronchitis:
10 drops Thyme and 5 drops Eucalyptus
or
10 drops Hyssop and 5 drops Eucalyptus
Asthma:
10 drops Rosemary, 10 drops Lavender and 5 drops Hyssop
Sinus Problems:
5 drops Lavender and 2 drops Peppermint
Arthritis:
10 drops Chamomile and 5 drops Sage
Blues (mild depression):
10 drops Rose and 10 drops Chamomile

Chapter Three
Perfume Blending
(Aromacology)

Perfume blending is the wonderful art of mixing complementary aromatics together to form one pleasing scent. Believed to have been started in ancient Egypt and carried on to the modern day, it is quite easy to produce your own personal scent. For this application of floral use you may utilize pure essential Aromatherapy oils and/or fragrance oils. There are hundreds and hundreds of essential oils and thousands of fragrance oils on the market so to simplify things a bit we will stay with aromatics derived from flowers and blends considered floral in nature.

Just as with the art of Aromatherapy, perfume use has a long and interesting history. Believed to be the first fragrance to incorporate modern day ingredients was Hungary Water which was prepared for Queen Elizabeth of Hungary in 1370. Some say that it was based on lavender and bergamot while others point to rosemary. Many stories swirl as to why she commissioned it or was given it by someone else as a gift but the fact remains that it was the first to use an alcohol solution to render it. After that period, people found that preparing perfumes in that manner was more cost effective and the fragrance had a better shelf life. In the Renaissance period the Italians perfected the art but throughout the 16th century France became masters in the world of fragrances for the whole of Europe.

One must remember that up until the concocting of Chanel number 5, all perfumes were made with real essential oils. Imitations were not an option so not only did the fragrances smell wonderful but they also disinfected and provided other healing qualities to the wearer. Unfortunately, when the use of perfume became extremely popular to the point of being farcical in the 17th and 18th century, bathing and personal hygiene were not. Add this to the lack of proper sewage systems and you have a disaster waiting to happen. Outbreaks of various, sometimes preventable diseases was an everyday occurrence and it wasn't much of a sight to see women, heavily powdered and perfumed strolling around with open, infected sores on their bodies. In an attempt to combat the sickening odors around them, fountains that normally spewed water were filled with perfume. The walls and drapes were splashed with fragrance and flowers both fresh and cut were used where ever possible. Perfumes were applied frequently throughout the day and clothing was scented with sachets and potpourris. Women would also carry with them a bouquet of flowers called a Nosegay, also known as a Tussie Mussies. The specially prepared bouquet of aromatic flowers and herbs were held close to the face while strolling the streets. In this modern day people tend to romanticize the heavy use of perfumes, colognes, etc., but in reality it was a way of life and some measure of protection from the widespread plagues and out-breaks of disease.

In the Victorian age, perfume was still an important part of life, especially for women. Intricate clocks were even made with a different scent or flower next to each hour. When the clock chimed or turned to the next hour the women of the house would change their perfume to the one associated to the new time of day or night. Women of that time were very intrigued and interested in anything that seemed exotic or came from the Orient. Perfumes and potpourris of that time reflect that and contain spices and exotic floras.

Today, the perfume industry uses essential oils and fragrance oils to formulate various fragrances. Unconventional scents such as human pheromones and chocolate are combined with age old ones to produce interestingly new yet many times familiar perfumes. Neroli, Jasmine and Rose are still the most used oils and you will find a hint of either or all in many of your favorite aromas. Preparing your own perfume as the professionals do isn't as hard as you think. Simply fol-low the system of combining complementary scents and notes. Most commercial perfumes include all three notes for a well rounded blend but some lighter scents only use top and middle notes. For the first time perfumer, keeping a fragrance blend simple is best. Use 2 or 3 oil scents at a time.

Oil note and Blending chart

Perfume blending is not hard and below is a chart to help you formulate your own, personal scent. Some essential Aromatherapy oils are quite expensive such as rose and jasmine. Others are totally unavailable such as in the case of cherry, etc., so fragrance oils can be used instead. Just like essential oils, fragrance oils should not be applied to the skin directly. Make sure to dilute your blend in a scentless base/carrier oil such as vegetable or almond first. You should note the scents each oil blends best with and compliments by looking at the note category it falls in. Top note oils dissipate faster from the skin and will be the first scent the nose detects in a blend. A middle note can be used to bridge the top and base note together. It is the second scent the nose detects and it lingers on the skin for a while longer than the top note. The base note rounds a blend out and is the last scent that is left on your skin when the top and middle have totally dissipated. It is also the last scent your nose will detect. Being mindful of note categories will help your blend to come out more well rounded.

Top Notes

Bergamot ....Jasmine, Lavender, Cypress, Neroli, Juniper
Lemon Verbena..........Palmarosa, lemon & most florals
Mandarin Orange ......Cloves, Rose, Ylang Ylang, Cinnamon
Petitgrain ....Geranium, Orange, Jasmine, Bergamot, Clove
Lemon ....Ylang Ylang, Juniper, Cedarwood, Lavendar
Lily of the Vally ....Musk, Violet, Sandalwood, Cedarwood
Neroli ....Clary sage, Rose, Violet, Lemon, Ylang Ylang
Lime ....Most florals & Citruses, Petitgrain, Rosemary
Orange ....Juniper, Cypress, Most spices, Ylang Ylang
Lemongrass...............Lavender, Rose, Juniper, Geranium
Sweet Pea ....Musk, Vanilla, Lemon Verbena
Peppermint..............Lavender, Rosemary, Marjoram
Cinnamon ....Rose, Violet, Myrrh, & most spices
Clove ....Rosemary, Peppermint

Middle Notes

Almond ....Vanilla, Rose, & Most spices
Peach ....Jasmine, Gardenia, Violet, Sandalwood
Pineapple ....Vanilla, Most fruits, Narcissus
Magnolia ....Honeysuckle, Musk, Sandalwood
Strawberry ....Gardenia, Jasmine, Violet, & Most fruits
Geranium ....Lavender, Bergamot, Lemon Grass
Carnation ....Heliotrope, Musk, Most spices & florals
Tuberose ....Geranium, Carnation, Rose, Petitgrain
Rosewood ....Blends with most oils including spices & florals
Narcissus...................Neroli, Heliotrope, Sandalwood
Violet ....Hyacinth, Tuberose, Clary sage & most florals
Mango ....Neroli, Vanilla, Begamot
Lavender...................Geranium, Pine, Orange & most florals
Neroli ....Rose, Jasmine, Ylang Ylang,Violet, Lavender
Cherry ....Vanilla, Almond, Most fruits
Chamomile...............Jasmine, Rose, Neroli, Geranium, Lavendar
Coconut ....Gardenia, Ylang Ylang, Vanilla

Frangipani ....Heliotrope, Rose, Nerolie
Marjoram ....Lavender, Rosemary, Cedarwood, Cypress
Gardenia...................Jasmine, Rose, Tuberose, Ylang Ylang
Honeysuckle ....Neroli, Musk, Sandalwood
Jasmine.....................Rose, Clary sage, Sandalwood, Strawberry
Lilac ....Rose, Violet, Heliotrope
Base Notes
Patcholi....................Rose, Lavender, Geranium, Cassia, Jasmine
Cinnamon ....Ylang Ylang, Rose, Violet, Myrrh
Balsam ....Jasmine, Rosewood, Manderin, Benzion
Cedarwood ....Jasmine, Hyacinth, Rose, Neroli, Rosemary
Clary sage ....Jasmine, Lavender, Geranium, Cypress
Myrrh......................Frankincense,Geranium, Lavender, Neroli
Vetiver ....Violet, Jasmine, Rose, Cassia, Ylang Ylang
Vanilla ....Jasmine, Neroli, Ylang Ylang, Patchouli
Heliotrope ....Neroli, Carnation, Violet & most florals
Musk ....Jasmine, Rose, Tuberose. Narcissus
Frankincense.............Lavender, Geranium, Neroli, Cinnamon
Black Papper.............Rosemary, Lavender, & most florals
Sandalwood ....Rose, Jasmine, Ylng Ylng

Other things that may be added to your perfume blend include flavor extracts of Vanilla, Coconut, even Chocolate. Being that these extracts are rendered in alcohol or other non-oil bases, they can separate from the oils in your perfume. Just remember to shake your scent well before using. Honey may be included in a blend to act as a natural fixative or gum of benzion may extend the life of your perfume. Remember though that these botanicals have their own scent and may change the entire fragrance for the better or worse. Crushed rose or other flower petals add interest as well as scent, over time, to a personal perfume blend.

Use pungent oils such as orange, black pepper, peppermint, lemon, etc., in smaller amounts so that your whole blend is not completely taken over. After the additions of each oil, be sure to incorporate it well and smell to see how your blend is progressing.

Perfume recipes:
Lavender Dream
10 drops Lavender
5 drops Vanilla
Exotic Spice
5 drops Neroli
5 drops Ylang Ylang

1 to 2 drops Cinnamon
Luscious Rose
10 drops Rose
3 to 4 drops Vanilla
1 to 2 drops Musk
Violet Moon
10 drops Violet
2 to 3 drops Musk
1 to 2 drops Honeysuckle
Antique Rose
10 drops Rose
2 to 3 drops Patchouli
2 to 3 drops Lavender
Exotic Gardenia
10 drops Gardenia
5 drops Coconut
1/8 to 1/4 teaspoon honey
Romantic Flower Garden
10 drops Lavender
2 drops Vanilla
5 drops Rose
1 to 2 drops cinnamon
Exotic Violet
10 drops Violet
3 drops Almond
3 drops Rose
1 drops Benzion
Honey Moon Drops
12 drops Honeysuckle
1 to 2 drops Vanilla
1/8 to 1/4 teaspoon honey
Cologne:
To make a great cologne with alcohol, combine 1/4 cup of spring water and 1/4 cup vodka. Add essential oils of choice and shake well. Let cure for a week before use. You can also soak fresh flower petals in the 1/4 cup of vodka for a week, in the refrigerator. After it has steeped, remove plant material and add 1/4 cup water. A little honey may be added to help preserve your cologne.

Perfumed Waters:

Simple add essential oil combination of choice to 1/2 to 1 cup of spring water. Add a little bit of honey and shake really well. This works best if placed in a dark colored glass spray bottle. Keep in the refrigerator in between use.

Hard Perfumes:

Add perfume combination of choice to:

4 Tablespoons sweet almond or vegetable oil

1/2 to 1 teaspoon bees wax

1/2 teaspoon natural honey

Heat all ingredients in a small sauce pan over very low heat or in a microwave safe cup placed in a microwave turned on medium to low setting. When everything is liquefied together, remove from heat and add perfume combination. Stir and pour into a clean container with a lid. Store in the refrigerator in between uses.

Modern Day Effleurage:

For a easy version of this age old method of perfume making, take 1 to 3 cups of flower petals and place them in a Mason jar with a lid. Pour 1 to 1 & 1/2 cup of a light oil such as sweet almond over the petals. Mix around with a spoon and cover tightly. Let cure for one week. Remove plant material and add a fixative such as benzion or a pinch of orrisroot powder.

Many confuse the art of perfume blending with Aromatherapy, which in reality differ in many ways. One of the largest being that Aromatherapy can only use pure essential oils for a healing effect. Perfume blending on the other hand, also known as Aromacology, can use either essential oils or fragrance oils. When you are making a synergistic blend with Aromatheray, you are predominately doing so to create a more effective, healing concoction. In the case of perfume blending, you are combining scents to create a pleasing effect, i.e. because they complement each other aromatically. Perfumes do not have the same powers of healing Aromatherapy does and any effect they have on the bodies system is related to the Olfactory portion of the brain and it's correlation to moods, memory recall, depression, etc., where as essential oils have the ability to penetrate the skin and remedy from within.

· Chapter Four ·
Dried Floral Use (Herbology)

Dried flowers are some of the easiest to use and render medicinally. Drying leaves, petals, etc., from your own garden or from out in the wild is quite simple as well. They can in turn be used as teas or prepared into tinctures. In this chapter we will be taking a step by step look at how to properly dry flowers for medicinal and ornamental/aromatic use.

Drying Flowers for Consumption and Aromatic Applications

The way you go about drying a plant, depends on what portion of it will be dried, i.e. root, flower, etc. Equipment you may need includes; a food dehydrator, a metal screen, paper towels, newspaper or another sort of absorbent paper, brown paper bags, kitchen shears/scissors, a wire coat hanger, string or cooking twine, clean glass or plastic bottles.

Drying Leaves

After harvesting the leaves from the plant, be sure to take care not to damage it in any way. Doing so can lead to loss of medicinal qualities in the form of the plants inherent essential oils. Wipe leaves off with a damp cloth if you need to remove loose dirt, sand, etc. Try not to over saturate the leaves with water or wash them fully. Also be sure to prepare the leaves in an area that is not near an open window or direct sunlight. If leaves are left on the steams, gather loose a couple plants and tie them together with the string. Hand them upside down and fasten them to a wire coat hanger. If you like, you can protect them by placing pieces of newspaper around the plants, loosely or you can put a paper bag with air holes cut into it over them and tie the open end closed. For leaves that have been removed from the stems or for drinking small quantities, you can lay out either a wire rack or cookie sheet. Cover with paper towels or absorbent materials and carefully spread leaves out. Give them enough room from each other and don't overlap which can lead to improper drying and mold growth.

The best places to dry your plants happens to be a closet or inside of your garden or tool shed. The area must be very well ventilated, very dry and dark to prevent mold growth and sunlight damage to plants. The temperature can be from 70 to 90 degrees Fahrenheit/ 20 to 32 Celsius. The drying process can be sped up a bit by installing a fan that blows fresh air over your drying leaves. Depending on the thickness of the leaves, the drying process can take anywhere from four days to a couple of weeks. Be sure to check them in-between that time to make sure they are drying properly and not harboring mold. If you see any signs of mold or mildew of any kind, discard at once. Leaves that are completely dry are brittle and crackly to the touch. They should appear duller and a bit paler than fresh leaves. Break leaves up into smaller pieces if need be and remove them from the stem of the plant if they were left on. Store in a clean container made of thick glass or plastic. Dark bottles work better than clear to prevent sun damage of contents. Be sure to continue to store your dried leaves/herbs in a dry, dark place to prevent mold from forming. Most dried leaves can be kept for up to 18 months, if stored properly.

Drying Flowers

You will find the steps for drying leaves pretty much the same for flower heads. For very tiny or delicate flowers such as lavender and baby's breath, you want to keep the whole plant intact while drying it. Do not attempt to remove the flowers because they will break and become damaged thereby releasing the medicinal qualities. Flowers that have a very large centers need to have the petals removed and dried. The centers can be discarded. If you are not planing on using the plant medicinally, you can keep the whole flower intact. When drying the heads only, lay them out on a paper covered cookie sheet or wire screen carefully and be sure to give each one as much room a possible. Don't layer them. Once dry, they should have retained most of their original color and be brittle to the touch. The drying process for flowers can take up to three weeks and like leaves, must be checked every once in a while for signs of mold. Store on a cookie sheet so that they are flat (if whole flower heads) preventing their petals from crumpling and breaking off.

Drying Roots

Unlike flowers and leaves, roots should be dried in an oven or food dehydrator. This is due to the fibrous of the root and all the moisture it contains. All dirt should be removed from the root along with the hairy off shoots. If the root is quite large, split it first in half and then proceed to cut it into small rounds or chunks. They then need to be placed in a very low oven. Rhizomes and some roots such as marshmallow should be peeled before drying. When completely dried, they will become somewhat brittle. Store in a clean container in a dark, dry environment. Some roots, once dried attempt to draw moisture out of the air, causing the root to become soft and grow mold. To help prevent this, make sure they are kept in a very cool and dry spot in your house and that their container has a airtight fitting lid.

Flowers that Retain Their Scent

Not all flowers retain their original scent, while others become more pungent over time. The following flowers work well for aromatic applications such as potpourris, sachets, etc.

Rose
Lavender
Orange blossoms
Thyme
Chamomile
Marigold
Elder flower
Rosemary
Lemon Verbena
Geranium
Lilac
Daisy
White Carnations
Baby's Breath
Whole Rose Buds
Honeysuckle
Violet
Freesia
Lily of the Valley

If you need a splash of color in your aromatic concoctions, these flowers best retain their color when dried.

Borage
Bee Balm
Daisy
Feverfew
Forget-me-not
Zannias
Poppy
Marigold

Ways of Using Your Dried Flowers, Leaves, Roots, etc.

Dried flowering plants can be used for many medicinal applications, just as herbs are. You can use a singular plant or you can make a combination which will create a synergistic effect. Remedies can be made for both internal and external use, quite easily.

Infusions:

Better known as a tea, infusions are a simple way of extracting the medicinal qualities out of leaves, flowers and other delicate parts of plants. Bring water to a boil and turn heat off. Pour the hot water over plant material which has been placed in another heat proof tea pot or kettle and let steep for a few minutes. Pour into cups, using a strainer, and serve. The same effect can be done with a tea ball or bags. Drink the tea hot or chill ed. Infusions can be used externally for certain skin conditions, such as acne and as an additive to bath water.

Decoctions:

Decoctions are used on plant material that doesn't yield it's healing qualities as easily as more delicate plants. This includes roots and stems which require boiling or simmering for a time. Instead of being ingested like tea, decoctions are usually turned into tonics, syrups and tinctures as their resulting taste is more than likely not very pleasant. Once made it can be stored in a tea cup or in larger quantities in the refrigerator. Just as with infusions, many external uses can be made from decoctions such as compresses, bath additives, etc.

Syrups:

To make a syrup you can either use natural honey or sugar. The honey method is easier as all you need to do is add 1 part honey to 1 part liquid infusion or decoction of the plant of your choice. You must heat the honey, stir in the liquid infusion or decoction, turn heat off and let it cool a bit before transferring to a clean glass bottle or ceramic cup. This method works well for botanicals that don't have pleasant tastes or that are very bitter. When preparing a syrup with honey, remember not to give it to toddlers or babies under the age of two.

Tinctures:

Tinctures are made by soaking botanicals in alcohol and thereby making a concentrated remedy. Simply place leaves, flowers, etc. of choice in a large glass container and pour over it with a high alcohol containing liquor such as Vodka or Rum. Do not use rubbing alcohol or anything that can not be ingested or may prove toxic. Put a tight fitting top/lid on the container and let it sit for about two to three weeks. Pick it up every once in a while and swish it around a bit. It should be stored in a cool, dark place where the sun can not get to it. When it's finished steeping, remove plant material by straining it well and place in a clean container. Store in the refrigerator.

Cold and Hot Infused Oils:

A great way of preparing wonderful massage or culinary oils is to use the hot or cold infusion method. It is very much like a normal infusion except quality oil is used instead of water. For the cold oil infusion, all you need to do is take a wide mouth jar and add plant matter of your choice. Pour oil, depending on it's finished application, over the botanicals and cover tightly. Instead of keeping it in a dark place, place it on a sunny spot so that the heat from the sun allows the oil draw out the plant's medicinal essential oils and vitamins. Let steep for up to three weeks. When done, use a piece of cheese cloth or a strainer to strain off all plant material. If you will be using it for a culinary oil, you can leave a bit of the bigger pieces of plant in if you like for interest. Keep refrigerated and sterilize the bottle that it will be going into if possible.

Hot oil infusions are also simple to prepare. Heat a large pot of oil on the stove, being sure there is no water on your hands, in the pot, etc. to cause it to pop and splatter. Be very careful to pour in botanicals of your choice. Stir to get all the plant material down into the oil and heat on extremely low heat for up to two hours. Once done, strain off plant material and pour into a clean, sterilized bottle. Keep refrigerated.

Cold and Hot Compress:

All you need to make a compress is to take some of the decoction or infusion you've made earlier and pour it into a bowl. Soak a cotton cloth in it for a few minutes and wring it out a bit. This cloth can now be placed over the forehead or on any other part of the body that needs relief. The liquid you soak the cloth in can be heated up in a microwave or a bit over low heat on the stove or it can be chilled for a cold compress. If using the hot compress method, you may need to keep re-soaking the cloth a few times as it cools after a few minutes.

Poultice:

A poultice is like a natural plant plaster that is kept on for longer periods than a compress. You can make a poultice in a few ways. If using dried herbs, you can pound them until they are a powder consistency and add a little water to form a paste. This can in turn be applied to the skin and left on for up to 30 minutes. You can also add the dried herbs to dried clay, add water to form a mask and apply. Either way you should cover your poultice with a light covering of gauze to prevent it from rubbing off onto anything. Use hot water for a hot poultice paste or ice water for a cold poultice.

Ointments:

Healing ointments are made with the infused cold or hot oil that you might have made earlier and a bit of stiffing agent such as natural bees wax. Petroleum jelly can also be use but I prefer bee's wax because it is much more natural, unrefined and contains no chemicals. Heat the oil in a small pot, add extra plant material if you like to you can just use the cold or hot infused oil as is, add bee's wax and stir until completely incorporated. If you added extra herbs, you will need to strain them off once the mixture has cooled down a bit. Pour your oil mixture into a clean glass or ceramic container and let it cool completely in the refrigerator. When done you will have a wonderful, smooth ointment that can be applied to the skin for protection from elements and to help heal.

Steam Inhalation:

Use a large bowl that has been filled with boiling or simmering water. Quickly add a couple tablespoons of dried plant material and place your face over the bowl. Cover your head with a large towel or cloth to help channel the steam towards you. Inhale with deep breaths as many times as possible. This works well for congestion problems.

Powders:

Powders can be made by chopping up dried herbs into small pieces and placing them into coffee grinder, small food processor or in a mortar and pestle. Pulverize into a fine powder and use in teas, on food or place in empty gelatin capsules for internal use. These powders can also be used externally as baths powders, soaps, etc.

Massage Oil:

A great way of making your own massage oil is to make an herbal color or hot infusion and add a few drops extra of essential oil of your choice. Sweet almond oil works best for massage use. Just before giving a massage, you can place a few drops, as a little goes a long way, and rub in-between the palms of the hands to warm. More can be applied later, if needed. This also works well for self massages.

Burning Them:

Certain dried flowers are wonderful when burned and emit a great scent throughout the house. People for thousands of years have been burning certain botanicals because of their believed healing or sacred nature. One of these were rosemary which was burned in households throughout history for driving away evil spirits and to protect the inhabitants from disease and the plague. You too can do this by buying a well made incense burner which is large, placing inside a lit clean burning charcoal disk, specially made for burning herbs and sprinkling the herbs of your choice over top. Follow the direction on the charcoal disk for lighting it. Not all flowers smell the same when burned so try these first.

Rose petals
Lavender
Rosemary
Thyme
Chamomile
Yarrow

You can combine all of these to make a special blend or experiment with other flowers to see what sort of fragrance, if any, that they emit. Remember to never leave smoldering herbs/flowers in the reach of children or unattended at any time. Doing so can lead to extremely dangerous situations. Keeping a small cup of water at hand doesn't hurt either in case a stray spark flies off and catches something near by on fire.

Chapter Five

Bach Flower Remedies

"Think of the patient, not the disease" was Dr. Edward Bach's motto. This aphorism embodies the healing thought behind Bach Flower remedies. In this healing method, flower tinctures are prepared and administered under the tongue to relieve the root of ailments which can be fear, anxiety, anger, etc., for example. It was Dr. Bach's thought that emotional issues lead to illness and that flower remedies, which are highly diluted, can safely be used to change these imbalances.

In order to find the correct remedy, you must analyze the way the person or you yourself feels, emotionally instead of the ailment or symptoms. Whether you have a high fever or the chills, you would be given the same remedy regardless, as long as your emotional state remained the same. Like Homeopathic medicine, the remedy is not taken to treat, cure or stop a symptom or illness. Instead, it is given to reverse sometimes negative emotional states which are harmful to the body and that lead to physical sickness.

Dr. Bach researched and found 38 key remedies derived from flowers accessible to him in England. After the late 1970's, more flower remedies were discovered and created using native plants of other locals, such as the America's and Australia. Almost any flower has the possibility of becoming a remedy with companies and institutes constantly researching to find more. Dr. Bach's original 38 are still the most used and the foundations for healing with flower remedies.

How to Prepare Your Own Remedy

You'll find it easy to make your own flower remedies. There are a few ways of going about it. One way can be likened to making a sun tea. This method works well for delicate flowers. Fresh, ripe flowers in their fullest bloom are picked early in the morning, preferably when covered in dew. Place the flowers in a large bowl filled with spring water and allow to sit, uncovered in a sunny window or in full sunlight outside for three hours. The flowers are then traditionally removed with a twig of the same plant so the flower water is not contaminated. Pour the flower water into a glass bottle which has been sterilized and make a ratio of 1 part flower water and 1 part alcohol. Brandy was traditionally used. This solution is call the *Mother Essence*. This is then diluted 50/50 in more Brandy. This acts as a natural preservative. A few drops of the mother essence is then added to more brandy and the whole batch is bottled and distributed. If you make this yourself, your tincture will be probably a bit more concentrated then those found in stores.

For flowers that don't yield their essences as easily, the decoction method is used. This works well on twigs, tougher tree leaves, etc. Place plant material in a small pan to pot and cover with spring water. Bring this to a boil and then turn heat off completely. Let steep and cool, then filter it through a sieve or Chinese hat. Mix with Brandy as above and the rest of the procedures are the same. One mother essence can produce many bottles of flower remedies. Remedies should be stored in a glass bottle which is dark brown or cobalt blue to prevent sunlight damage. Tops/lids should be twisted on very tightly and bottles should be refrigerated if at all possible.

Ways of Using Bach Flower Remedies

There are many ways of using these remedies so incorporating their use into your daily life isn't that difficult. Most flower remedies can be found in health food stores in tincture form. They are suspended in alcohol and traditionally a few drops are placed under the tongue for on the spot treatment. If you need to give a remedy to someone who can not tolerate alcohol, (such as a baby or small child), you can add the drops to any liquid beverage such as warm or chilled tea, fruit or vegetable juice, or even water. Make sure to stir it in well. Flower remedies can also be used externally. One drop can be rubbed onto the temples, the back of the knees, behind the ears, and at any of the pulse points. Another way of using Bach flower remedies is to place the solution into a spray bottle and mist around your head and face, breathing in deeply to take the vapors in.

Bach Flower Remedy Table

The key to using flower remedies is to pick one that is indicated for the emotion that you are feeling right at that moment or over an extended amount of time.

Agrimony ....Hiding mental torture behind a fake cheerful persona.

Aspen ....Fear of unknown things that are about to or might happen to you.

Beech..............................Intolerance, constant negative feelings towards others.

Centaury ....The inability to say 'no', the neglecting of yourself to aid others needs.

Cerato ....Lack of trust in one's own decisions, asking for others advice constantly.

Cherry Plum ....Fear of losing your mind, controlling your impulses.

Chestnut Bud	Failure to learn from mistakes, repeating mistakes over and over.
Chicory	Selfishness, possessive of love ones time and affection.
Clematis	Dreaming of the future instead of concentrating on present projects.
Crab Apple	Shame over deeds you know you should not have done, self-hatred.
Elm	Overwhelmed by responsibility, overextending yourself with work.
Gentian	Unable to start over again after a setback, discouraged after a setback.
Gorse	Hopelessness and despair on overcoming an illness.
Heather	Self-centered and self-concern, feeling that others are not listening.
Holly	Envy and jealousy, constant suspicions of others motives.
Honeysuckle	Living in the past, wishing constantly to relive your life over again.
Hornbeam	Procrastination, too tired to start projects at work and at home.
Impatiens	Impatience of people and things that don't move at your speed.
Larch	Lack of confidence, lack of trying new things in fear of failing.
Mimulus	Phobias of certain things around you.
Mustard	Deep gloom and depression for seemingly no reason.
Oak	Throwing yourself into your work/project to the point of exhaustion.
Olive	Exhaustion following mental or physical effort, illness.
Pine	Guilt over others mistakes, wishing you could do a better job at work.
Red Chestnut	Over concern for the health and safety of loved ones.
Rock Rose	Terror and panic, constant nightmares.
Rock Water	Self-denial, feeling you must live up to a set ideal.
Scleranthus	Inability to choose between alternatives, extreme mood swings.
Star of Bethlehem	Shock, personal loss that you have failed to recover from.
Sweet Chestnut	Feeling that there is nothing to live for, impending doom.
Vervain	Over enthusiasm for justice that must be done.
Vine	Must have complete control over others around you.

Walnut ....Having problems making changes in one's life and letting go of the past.

Water Violet ....Pride and aloofness, wishing to spend time alone constantly.

White Chestnut...............Constant mental arguments, problems sleeping because of worries.

Wild Oat........................Uncertainty over one's direction in life, feeling that life is passing by.

Wild Rose ....Apathy, not bothering to change the environment around you to bring joy to your life.

Willow ....Self-pity, a constant feeling that others around you have done you wrong.

The above is a condensed table. Dr. Bach believed in looking at the persons emotional state closely and asking questions to determine the correct remedy to prescribe and use. Remedies are to be used over a period of time which can last up to two weeks. If a real improvement isn't seen in a reasonable amount of time, seek the attention of a medical physician. Once again, flower remedies are meant to treat the underlying emotional sate which may be causing a particular condition, not the condition itself directly. If the underlying feelings are taken care of, other problems associated with them will be relieved. Flower remedies work well for extended use and because of their dilute nature, are safe to take over a long span of time.

· Chapter Six ·

Secret Flower Recipes

In this chapter you will find wonderful recipes that are easily prepared using simple ingredients along with flowers in essential oil, dried and fresh form. Before making a product using any type of flower, make sure it has been grown organically and is free of all pesticides and pollutants. If you can, grow your own flowers or make sure the flowers you buy say organically grown. If wildcrafting or picking flowers in the woods, etc. be sure that the area has not been treated with pesticides or other chemicals. Many park systems do this so check before picking anything first. Also stay clear of gathering flowers from the roadside. Chemicals build up on the leaves and petals of such plants because of exhaust from the constant passage of cars and other vehicles. When using flowers for medicinal purposes it is always important to use the finest quality available.

Plants such as dandelion, violet, clover, etc., are pretty easy to find growing in the wild and are for the most part not hybrids. On the other hand flowers such as roses are many times hybrids and therefore can not be used therapeutically. This can be due to the lack of scent or growth of rose hips. The petals can also lack certain vitamins and nutrients found in wild varieties. If you are familiar with flower gardening, you will be able to tell which plants you are growing or choosing are hybrids and which are classic species. Most wild flowers have smaller blossoms than their hybrid counterparts. Color can also be an indicator as well. Flower petals which contain a noticeable pattern or bright hue are many times bred that way. The key is to look for flowers that retain their inherent scent, foliage and wild appearance.

Doing a Patch

It is always wise, especially with products made with natural botanicals, to do a patch test first before applying to suggested areas. Before using any of the remedies included in this book, I strongly suggest doing so for the following reasons: 1.) You may be unknowingly allergenic to one or more of the botanical ingredients. 2.) You may have very sensitive skin that reacts differently to the fresh product versus the dried product. 3.) The nutrients in the fresh botanical product is many times stronger than the same found in commercial blends.

Doing a patch test is very simple. Apply a small portion of the product to the skin found on the inside of your arm. This may sound like a strange area but it happens to be where the skin is most sensitive. Leave on for 24 hours or overnight to determine if you will develop a reaction. If no irritation appears then you may proceed with using the concoction. If any sign of tenderness or rash occurs discontinue use at once and if it persists contact a medical professional such as a dermatologist. All of the recipes have been tested in some shape or form by me personally but I can not guarantee your skin will react the same as mine does. One must always use a sound mind when making products to apply to the skin or hair.

Equipment Needed

The following is a list of items you will find helpful when making your floral concoctions:

A blender or food processor

A strainer (Chinese hat)

Pieces of cheese cloth or other fine, pores fabric

String (used to tress meats and poultry works best)

Wire or natural fiber whisk

Small sauce pan or pot

Measuring spoons and cups used for dry and wet ingredients

Bowls of assorted sizes

Small metal or wooden spoons for mixing

Small glass or plastic bottles and containers

Eye dropper

Glass Sterilization

If you are preparing concoctions that contain a large quantity of oil or water, I would recommend sterilizing the glasses first if that will be what you will be using as a container. This can help prevent mold growth and contamination from botulism. All you need to do is immerse the glass bottles in water and turn heat on medium to high. Bring to a boil and turn heat off. Pour recipe right into warm bottles and let cool. Store in the refrigerator to help improve shelf-life.

Recipes for the Body and Bath:

Using essential oils and fresh flowers for body care and bath items is a real treat and can be quite simple. Most of the items, unless noted otherwise should be refrigerated and kept for no longer then a week. The longer the product sits, the more likely the active ingredients will dissipate and the overall concoction will become less effective. Remember to use the freshet ingredients possible and real Aromatherapy grade essential oils.

Vanilla Rose Body Oil:

4 Tablespoons olive oil

4 Tablespoons sweet almond oil

1 teaspoon pure vanilla extract

1 Cup fresh or 1/2 Cup dried rose petals

5 drops rose essential oil (optional)

Place oils and rose petals into a clean glass bottle. Let stand in your refrigerator for one week. After that period of time, strain off plant material and add vanilla and essential oil. Mix well before using as the vanilla may tend to separate. If you like, you can use essential oil of vanilla.

Basic Massage Oil:

1/4 Cup sweet almond oil

2 Tablespoon olive oil

1/2 teaspoon cocoa butter (optional)

Combine and heat ingredients until warm. Add either essential oil or plant matter of choice. You can add up to 15 drops of pure essential oil or 2 Tablespoons of dried or fresh leaves, petals, etc. If using the latter, let plant material steep in hot oil for 5 to 10 minutes, depending on desired strength. Strain oil through a sieve and place into a clean, sterilized bottle. Store in the refrigerator in between uses. The blends for perfumes in chapter three may be used to scent the massage oil or single notes of essential oils such as lavender, rose, geranium, etc. You will find these particular massage oils perfect for after bath moisturizing.

Honey Rose Body Oil:

4 Tablespoons sweet almond oil

1 teaspoon corn oil

2 Tablespoons olive oil

1/2 teaspoon natural honey

5 drops essential oil of rose

1 to 2 teaspoons vitamin E oil

1 teaspoon powdered rose petal (optional)

To prepare powdered rose petal, first dry them as you would for use in potpourri. Using a small coffee grinder or mortar and pestle pulverize into a fine powder. Store in a tin container in a cool, dark place until ready to use. Discard if any mold appears. Mix all ingredients together and heat for a couple of seconds in the microwave to help everything to blend together. Store in the refrigerator in between use. This formula works excellently to help soften rough patches of skin such as on the elbows and knees. Apply as often as you like. The vitamin E and honey will help act as natural preservatives so this body oil will have a longer shelf-life. Discard if any signs of rancidity forms which can be detected by a strong odor not related to the aromatic floral extraction's.

Violet All Over Body Silk:

6 Tablespoons olive oil

1 teaspoon corn oil

1/4 teaspoon natural honey

1/4 teaspoon natural beeswax

1/4 Cup dried or 1/2 cup fresh violet flowers and leaves

Heat first four ingredients in a small pot or sauce pan. When beeswax has melted and oil is hot add dried or fresh violet. Stir constantly with a metal spoon. The fresh plant material may seem like too much at first but once it gets heated and starts to absorb the oil, it will wilt down. Turn heat off, cover pot and let steep 20 to 30 minutes. Strain off plant material and place in a clean, sterilized glass jars. Plastic will also do. Keep refrigerated in between uses. The beeswax will help the oils and honey solidify. If you would like a harder salve, add more beeswax. If you can find it, a few drops of violet essential oil is a great addition.

Floral Body Drenchers:

Floral waters are quite simple to make and use as body mists. Simple place dried or fresh flower of choice in 2 to 4 cups of spring water. Bring water to a boil and then turn heat down and let simmer for 5 minutes. Turn heat completely off and cover. Let steep for 10 to 20 minutes. The longer it sits in the water, the stronger the scent and medicinal qualities will become. Once finished steeping, strain through a sieve if you don't mind some plant matter left in or with a paper coffee filter and place into a cleaned, sterilized glass container and store in the refrigerator. You can also use a method of making "sun teas" to make your floral waters. Add flowers and essential oil to water placed in a glass jar or bottle which is clear. Set in a sunny window sill or area on the porch/deck. This method can take anywhere from one to seven days depending on the plant(s) being used. To apply, either put in a air-pump spray bottle and use it to mist yourself frequently or use it as an all over body splash right after a shower. Both ways are quite refreshing. The making and use of floral waters dates back to ancient Egypt, Greek and Roman eras. Depending on the type of flower you chose, these waters can be quite beneficial to the healing of skin disorders such as acne, psoriases, eczema, etc. Pour a cup or two into your next bath for an added treat or mix in a few teaspoons of dried clay powder to make a wonderful mask.

The various uses for these floral waters are enormous!

Natural Lavender Bath Powder:

1/2 Cup cornstarch

1/2 Cup rice flour

1/4 cup dried lavender flowers which has been ground or pulverized

3 drops lavender essential oil

Grind lavender to a fine powder consistency. Add it to the flour and cornstarch, making sure to mix well. Add a few drops of essential oil such as benzoin to act as a natural preservative. Store in a tin or plastic container and let cure for one week in the refrigerator. Being that this is made from natural ingredients, it is best to store it in the refrigerator to prolong the shelf-life. Perfect for after bath dusting in the evening as this recipe has the added bonus of helping you get a good nights sleep. Once again you can use this same recipes with any of the perfume recipes in chapter three to concoct your own personal scent collection.

Silky Ylang Ylang Powder:

1 & 1/2 Cup cornstarch

5 drops ylang ylang essential oil

1 teaspoon sweet almond oil or any extremely light oil such as jojoba

Mix all ingredients together using a blender or sealing plastic bag. Both ways will give equal results. Empty into a clean container and let cure 5 to 7 days so that scent mingles with the cornstarch. If you like, you can add a few teaspoons of orris root powder to act as a natural preservative. This is an excellent recipe for people with dry skin. The added oil will help moisturize and calm the skin. Great for use in the morning or anytime.

Geranium Deodorant Powder:

1 Cup cornstarch

2 Tablespoons baking powder

1 teaspoon orris root (optional)

5 to 10 drops geranium essential oil

Mix all ingredients well in a blender or by using a sealing plastic bag and the shake method. Empty into a clean container and let cure 5 to 7 days. Store in the refrigerator to help keep it fresh. Use a large powdered sugar shaker to dispense if you like. Very gentle yet very effective. Geranium essential oil is a great deodorant along with the baking soda. You can sprinkle this in your shoes and on your bedding as well. It's not simply covering over the odor with a perfume but neutralizing it, so it is important that you use a quality geranium essential oil and not a fragrance oil which is pure synthetic scent.

Variation:

Peppermint Foot Powder:

Instead of the geranium essential oil add peppermint and ground peppermint leaves which are easily made in a small coffee grinder. Mix everything well and let cure for a week. This works well rubbed on the ankles and soles of the feet to help deodorize as well as sprinkled anywhere that needs the energizing scent of real peppermint!

Petal Soaps:

Making your own floral soaps are simple when you use pre-made soap and dried flowers.

Fill a small pot with cold water and bring it to a fast simmer. Using a plastic zip lock bag, place glycerin soap which has been cubed into small chunks inside and close the top. Place this bag into another plastic, self closing bag and tie it closed. Place bag in simmering water and dip and move it around until the soap has melted. As soon as it has, remove the bag from the water and wipe the outside of the bag off well. Just like with melting chocolate, getting water into the soap will ruin it. Take a small tea box and line it with tin foil. Spray a little cooking oil inside if you like. If you don't want to use a tea box you can buy a special molds made for soaps from most craft stores or places that sell Aromatherapy products. Pour half of your soap, as soon as possible into the lined tea box. Sprinkle what ever flower petals you like onto the layer of soap. If they are larger, whole flower heads, take a tooth pick and push them down into the soap layer. Pour the rest of the hot, melted soap over the first later and leave the box in a well ventilated, dry, area. The heat in the soap will help draw out the medicinal and aromatic attributes of the herbs you added.

Essential oils can also be included in your soaps by adding it to the bag that the soap chunks are melted in. This way they are observed into the hot soap. Use the Aromatherapy or perfume blending charts to determine which combinations work best.

After your soap has cooled completely, take a warm knife with a little oil on it and slide your large block of floral soap into bars. Wrap the bars tightly in tissue paper and let them cure for up to a week.

Variation:

Mosaic Petal Soaps:

To make interesting mosaic soaps, simply take pre-made floral white soaps that are too small to be used anymore and cut them into small cubes or chunks. Don't use glycerin soaps because they will melt and not give the same effect you want, use a creamy white soap. Pour some melted glycerin soap into the bottom of the lined tea box and then add the cubed white or Castill soap and flower petals. Use a tooth pick to push them down and then pour more glycerin soap over top. Prepare as above.

Mosaic soaps are wonderful because they are unusual and you can use commercial, non-glycerin soap for the interesting effect. If you want your mosaic soap to be deep cleansing use oatmeal soap cubes or for softening your skin, use lavender soap cubes.

Rose Bath Oil:

1/2 Cup vegetable or sweet almond oil

20 drops rose essential oil

1/4 cup fresh or dried rose petals

1/4 teaspoon natural, pure honey (optional)

Combine all ingredients into an open mouth glass bottle and let sit in your refrigerator for about 1 week. After it has cured, remove rose petals and store in the refrigerator in-between uses. To use, add a couple tablespoons to hot bath water and enjoy. Works well on very dry skin conditions and in the winter time.

Peach Rose Bubble Bath

5 drops peach fragrance oil

10 drops rose essential oil

1/4 cup dried rose petals (optional)

1 bar natural glycerin soap

1/4 to 1/2 cup rose water

Melt soap as described for making Petal Soaps. Place rose petals, essential and fragrance oils into the bottom of a wide mouth glass jar. Pour in rose water and then add hot, melted soap. Place a top on the jar and shake the mixture well. It will thicken as the soap cools. Store in the refrigerator in-between uses. Add a couple tablespoon under hot running water to use. May also be used as a delicate body wash.

Recipes for the Complexion and Special Beauty Treatments:

There are many traditional recipes which include flowers as their base ingredient for beautifying the complexion and skin. Many ancient cultures believed creating concoction containing flowers, which were lovely to look at, would transfer their beauty to the human using it. While this may or many not be true, many flowers, especially rose and lavender can do wondrous things for the skin, including reducing fine lines and clearing up acne. Before trying of the recipes below, remember to do a patch test! The skin of the face can be very sensitive, especially when raw botanicals are used.

Age Defying Oil

2 Cups fresh calendula flowers

1 Cup olive oil

4 teaspoons of vitamin E oil

Place flowers in oil and allow to steep in the refrigerator for a few days. Strain off botanical matter and apply oil to the whole face or where lines appear twice a week.

Rose Milk Complexion Mask
1/4 Cup of whole milk
1/4 Cup heavy cream (optional)
10 drops essential oil of rose
1/2 teaspoon vanilla extract (optional)

Combine all ingredients well and apply to the entire face, paying special attention to avoid the eye area, and allow to dry on the face for 15 to 30 minutes. Store any remaining mask in the refrigerator no longer than a week. This mask can also be applied to other parts of the body such as the shoulders, knees, elbows, etc.

Petal Mask
1/4 Cup fresh rose petals
1 teaspoon dried lavender or lavender tea
2 drops rose essential oil (optional)
2 drops lavender essential oil (optional)
1 whole egg beaten
1 teaspoon fresh lemon juice or pure lemon extract
1 teaspoon vanilla extract
2 Tablespoon dried milk powder

Combine all ingredients in a small bowl and stir 50 strokes or until completely combined. Allow to rest in the refrigerator for 10 minutes and then spread over the entire face, paying special attention to avoid the eye and mouth area, and neck if enough remains. Leave on for about 15 to 20 minutes and then rinse off with warm water. Apply a moisturizing treatment afterwards. This mask not only smells heavenly, but will firm the skin wonderfully and really leave it smooth. Some like to use this as a hand treatment as well.

Rose Hip Buttermilk Mask
1/2 Cup rose hips crushed
1/4 Cup spring water
1/4 Cup buttermilk
2 Tablespoons dried milk powder
2 drops rose essential oil (optional)

Bring water to a boil and quickly add rose hips, being sure to turn heat off right after. Allow to steep until water is cooled. Strain off rise hips and add buttermilk and milk powder. To achieve a thicker mask, add more milk powder to get the consistency you want. Apply to the entire face, being sure to avoid the eye area. Allow to stay on up to 30 minutes. Rinse with warm water.

Elder Flower Complexion Elixir
1/2 Cup dried elder flower blossoms

1 Cup spring water

2 drops lavender essential oil (optional)

Pour boiling water over dried elder flowers and allow to steep until water is cool. Strain off plant matter and add lavender oil if it will be used. Place liquid in a glass bottle with a tight fitting lid and store in the refrigerator in-between use. Apply by soaking a washcloth in the elixir and gently going over the entire face with it in a circular pattern.

Chamomile Eye Elixir

1 black tea bag

1/3 Cup spring water

4 Tablespoon dried chamomile flowers

2 drops essential oil of Roman chamomile

Bring water to a boil and add tea and chamomile flowers. Turn heat off and allow tea to steep for about 15 minutes or until cooled. Strain off botanical matter and add essential oil. Place in a glass container and store in the refrigerator in-between use. To use, soak a cotton ball in the solution and apply around the eye area, in and inward motion starting from the edge of the eye and working in towards the nose. Leave in for 5 minutes and then rinse off gently with warm water.

Clarifying Oil

4 Tablespoons of violet flowers

4 Tablespoons sage

5 Tablespoons almond or jojoba oil

3 capsules of vitamin E oil

2 drops lavender essential oil (optional)

Combine all ingredients and allow to steep in the refrigerator for 1 to 2 weeks. Be sure to shake or stir the mixture everyday. Once cured, apply oil to the skin using a cotton ball. This is very good for clearing skin conditions such as minor acne and helping the skin to heal faster reducing scaring. May also be used on the lips to help stop cold sores from forming.

Rose Facial Moisturizer

1/3 teaspoon vegetable shortening

1 teaspoon jojoba or sweet almond oil

2 teaspoons fresh lemon juice

5 drops rose essential oil

1 teaspoon dried rose petals (optional)

In a small pot or double boiler over low heat, and combine all ingredients. Heat until liquefied. Remove from the heat and pour into a small container. Allow to set in the refrigerator. Apply to the face, paying special attention to dry skin areas.

Floral Facial Gel

1 teaspoon dried lavender or lavender tea

4 drops lavender essential oil (optional)

1/2 Cup aloe vera gel

1 teaspoon chamomile tea

1 teaspoon calendula tea

Combine all ingredients and place in a microwave proof container and heat in the microwave for about 1 or 2 minutes or until liquefied. Allow to cool slightly and strain off plant material if you like. Place in the refrigerator to set completely. Use on entire face as an evening or morning treatment.

Floral Recipes for Hair:

There are many floral botanicals which can nourish and bring life back to stressed out tresses! Essential oils also can be used with great success, especially in commercially bought products, as only a few drops are needed to enhance the product. Rosemary and chamomile are two of the most useful botanicals for the scalp and hair and may be used in either herbal or essential oil form.

Natural Chamomile Shampoo

1/2 Cup soapwort (sweet William)

1/4 Cup chamomile flowers

1 teaspoon commercial, non-scented shampoo (optional)

2 drops chamomile essential oil (optional)

2 Cups spring or rain water

Bring water to a boil and pour over combined ingredients of soapweed, chamomile and shampoo. Let steep until mixture turns an amber color. Keep refrigerated in be-tween use. Being that it contains less detergent than probably what your used to with commercial products, you may need to leave the mixture on you hair for up to 15 minutes and then rinse out. This shampoo will not only clean but also give a wonderful herbal treatment each time you use it. Chamomile does have the power to lighten hair so, if you would like to maintain your lovely dark tresses, use rosemary instead.

Lavender Shampoo

1/2 Cup commercial, non-scented shampoo

1/3 Cup spring water

4 Tablespoon dried lavender or lavender tea

5 drops lavender essential oil (optional)

Bring water to a boil and pour over dried lavender. Allow to steep for up to 15 minutes. Strain off dregs and add liquid to soap and essential oil mixture. Place in a large glass container with a lid and shake well. May need to be stirred or shaken before each use.

Natural Hair Color for Blondes
1/2 Cup dried chamomile flowers
5 drops chamomile essential oil
Juice of 1 & 1/2 lemon
1/2 teaspoon pure lemon extract (optional)
1/2 Tablespoon lemon zest (peel)
4 Cups spring water

Bring water to a boil and pour over combined ingredients. Stir and allow to steep for 15 minutes. Strain off plant material and soak your hair in this concoction for at least 20 minutes. You may also pour the mixture over your hair repeatedly for 20 minutes. Rinse well from hair and allow hair to air dry, preferably in the sun. Honey, beer or white wine vinegar may also be added to the colorant.

Natural Hair Color for Redheads
1/2 Cup calendula (marigold) flowers
1 teaspoon carrot essential oil (optional)
1 Tablespoon pure cherry extract (optional)
2 Tablespoons red wine vinegar (optional)
2 Cups spring water

Follow directions as for the Natural Hair Color for Blondes.

Natural Hair Color for Brunettes
1/2 Cup dried rosemary
1 teaspoon translucent henna powder (optional)
5 drops rosemary essential oil (optional)
3 black tea bags
1 Cup prepared black coffee or espresso

Follow directions for the Natural Hair Color for Blondes. Black strap molasses may also be added for extra conditioning and highlights.

Natural Highlights for White Hair
3 Tablespoons translucent henna powder
10 drops Roman blue chamomile essential oil
1 Cup spring water

Follow directions for Natural Hair Color for Blondes.

Petal Hair Treatment
1/2 Cup fresh rose petals
5 drops rose essential oil
1/2 Tablespoon rose water flavoring extract (optional)
1 egg beaten
1/4 Cup white rum

Heat the rum and add the rose petals. Allow to cool and steep overnight. The next day, remove the plant material and add the beaten egg, extract and essential oil. Beat with a whisk well. 1/4 cup of water may also be added at this time. Apply to hair, paying special attention to the ends and leave on up to 30 minutes. Rinse off well with shampoo. Extra conditioning isn't needed afterwards.

Recipes for Common Problems:

For minor or non-life threatening, chronic conditions, flowers can be quite beneficial. Concoctions can be made quickly and used in various ways to help relieve the condition. Unless indicated otherwise these remedies should be stored in the refrigerator and kept cool as they have little or no preservative added to them and may spoil as a result.

Insomnia

Chamomile Apple Tea

Dried chamomile flowers, loose or bagged

Dried apply rings

Honey to taste

Bring water to a boil and turn heat off. Add apple rings and tea, cover and let steep for 5 minutes. Take 1 to 2 tea cupfuls before retiring to bed. The left over cooked apple rings may be given to children before bed if they do not want to drink the tea.

Coughs

Coltsfoot Tea

1/4 cup dried cultsfoot

1/4 cup dried chamomile

Honey to taste

Combine both herbs and make a simple infusion. Drink up to 3 teacup fulls a day for relief of minor coughs. This may also be turned into a syrup for a more coating, soothing effect. Fresh honeysuckle flowers may be added to the blend for extra cough relief.

Colds and Flu

Lavender Bath Bag

1/2 cup dry or 1 cup fresh lavender

1/4 cup dried milk

5 drops lavender essential oil

2 drops eucalyptus essential oil

1 piece of cheese cloth

Mix all ingredients together and place inside of a square of cheese cloth. Bring the four corners together and tie off at the top. Run a very hot bath and place the bath bag under the running water. Let water cool to a comfortable temperature and squeeze the bath bag a couple of times to extract all the healing qualities. The vapors from the lavender and eucalyptus will do wonders for helping your cough, congestion and more. This same bag may be used, without the dried milk for inhalation purposes only. Do this by placing it in a large bowl of hot, steaming water and cover your head with a towel.

Sprains
Soothing Compress
10 drops lavender essential oil
1/2 cup chamomile tea
1 washcloth
Combine essential oil and tea together and place in the refrigerator. Soak washcloth in the solutions and place on injured area(s). This solution may also be placed on a clean dry cloth pad to cover the effected area and then wrapped gauze to keep it in place.

Sunburn
Lavender Gel
1/4 cup alovera gel
10 drops lavender essential oil
1/2 to 1 teaspoon of vitamin E
Mix all ingredients together well and refrigerate for a few minutes if possible. Spread over burned areas being sure to use enough. This will help prevent blistering and promote the skin to rejuvenate faster. Apply as needed.

St. John's Wort Salve
1/2 cup dried St. John's Wort
1 teaspoon vitamin E
1 teaspoon vitamin A (optional)
1/4 teaspoon natural honey
6 tablespoons sweet almond or another base oil
1 teaspoon natural beeswax
1 dropper full of tincture of St. John's Wort, non-alcohol based (optional)
In a small pot combine oils and herbs, being sure to cover the pot with a lid and turning heat very low. Let cook until herbs are wilted and appear crispy. Let cool slightly and remove plant material through a sieve. Place back on the stove and add beeswax. Turn heat off after wax has melted and add honey and the tincture. Pour into a clean glass container and let cool in the refrigerator. This is extremely soothing as it stays on the top of the skin and makes a barrier from further irritation and skin damage due to clothing, etc. If St. John's Wort is unavailable, use calendula (marigold) flowers instead.

Sunburn Bath Treatment
5 black tea bags
1/4 cup dried lavender
2 cups oatmeal
5 drops lavender essential oil
Cheese cloth

Mix all ingredients together well, except tea and place into the center of a square of cheese cloth or another porous cloth. Add teat bags last, laying them on top. Close to form a pouch by bringing the corners together and tying it off with a piece if string/twine. Run a very hot bath and place bathe bag in water. Let water come to a comfortable temperature and squeeze bath bag a few times before entering. Works best if used right after a sunburn.

After Bath Rose Treatment
1/4 Cup rose water
1/4 Cup fresh lemon juice
1/4 Cup glycerin
3 capsules of vitamin E oil

Combine and place in a bottle. Shake well before applying to effected area with a cotton ball. Keep in the refrigerator no longer than a weeks time.

Insect Bites

Mosquito and Bee Gel
1 or 2 crushed chewable vitamin C tablets
1/4 cup alovera gel
10 drops lavender essential oil

Mix together all ingredients well and chill in the refrigerator for a few minutes if possible. Apply as needed to effected areas. This will help with swelling and itching. If you are highly allergic to bee stings, seek medical help immediately and use this as a follow up treatment. If you store this gel in a container with a tight fitting lid, it will keep in the refrigerator for a couple of months.

Mosquito Paste
5 drops chamomile essential oil
3 drops lavender essential oil
3 tablespoons baking soda

Combine all ingredients in a small cup and add warm water to make a thick paste. Spread paste on mosquito bites to take away the soreness, swelling and help prevent itching of the area. The lavender will also help the bite from becoming infected and causing scaring. This paste may also be used for other dermal irritants such as poison ivy, oak, etc.

Swollen Feet

Geranium Foot Bath

2 tablespoons baking soda

5 to 7 drops geranium essential oil

Pour hot water into a large basin and add above ingredients. Soak feet for 10 to 20 minutes. If you're feet are swollen from a condition such as diabetes, this treatment is not recommend. Over worked, tired feet will also benefit from this treatment.

Cellulite

Geranium Gel

1/2 cup alovera gel

10 to 12 drops geranium essential oil

5 drops lavender essential oil

2 drops orange essential oil (optional)

Mix together ingredients well and store in a clean, glass container in the refrigerator. Massage and work into the effected areas. This along with a proper diet and exercise may really work to tone and reduce the dimpled, loose look of cellulite effected skin.

Acne

Lavender Garlic Treatment

4 teaspoons vitamin E

1 tablespoon sweet almond or jojoba oil

5 drops lavender essential oil

3 cloves of fresh garlic

Slice garlic finely and add to oils. Place in a glass bottle and store in the refrigerator to cure for one week. Dab on effected areas only and let stay on over night. The smell is quite strong so only use at night. Aside from that this is quite a beneficial treatment for both adult and adolescent acne.

Bad Breath

Angelica Mouth Wash

2 Cups spring water

4 Tablespoon Angelica Seeds

Allow seeds to steep in boiling water for 30 minutes or until water is cool. Strain off seeds and place in a glass container with a tight fitting lid. Store in the refrigerator in-between use.

Floral Culinary Delights

Flowers were frequently used in Victorian dishes and still can be used to add not only color and interest but taste and nutrients as well. While not all flowers are edible and some are poisonous even, the below chat is provided for a reference of traditionally edible flowers. These flowers are also frequently used in tea blending to add taste. It is always wise, when cooking with flowers, to grow your own. This way you know that no pesticides were used and that they are completely organic. One should never attempt to use flowers from a florist as they are treated with a many toxic chemicals and even wildcrafting can be iffy. The best method is to cultivate your own flower garden according to a strict organic protocol and harvest them as needed.

Edible Flower Chart

Angelica
Anise Hyssop
Apple Blossoms
Arugula
Basil
Bee Balm
Borage
Burnet
Calendula
Carnation
Chamomile
Chicory
Chive Flowers/Buds
Chrysanthemum
Clover
Coriander
Cornflower
Dandelion
Day Lily
Dill
English Daisy
English Primrose
Fennel
Fuschia
Gardenia
Gladiolus
Hibiscus
Hollyhock
Honeysuckle
Hyssop
Impatiens

Jasmine
Johnny-Jump-Up
Lavendar
Lemon Blossom
Lemon Verbena
Lilac
Mallow
Marigold
Marjoram
Mint
Nasturium
Orange Flowers
Pansy
Peach Flowers
Pea Flowers
Pineapple Guava
Pineapple Sage
Radish
Redbud
Rose Petals and Hips
Rosemary
Runner Bean
Safflower
Scented Geranium
Snapdragon
Society Garlic
Squash Blossom
Strawberry Flowers
Sunflower
Thyme
Tuberous Begonia
Tulip
Violet
Yucca

NOTE: Asthmatics or others who suffer adverse allergic reactions to composite-type flowers such as calendula, chicory, chrysanthemum, daisy, English daisy, and marigold should be on alert for possible allergic reaction. Anyone whom is very sensitive to flowers should avoid culinary use of them.

Deserts:

Lavender Pound Cake

1 & 1/4 Cups all purpose white flour
3/4 Cup butter
3/4 Cup white sugar
3 eggs
4 to 5 Tablespoons dried lavender
1 teaspoon pure vanilla extract
1 teaspoon pure rose water extract (optional)
1/2 teaspoon lemon zest (peel)
1/4 teaspoon baking powder
1/4 teaspoon salt

Preheat your oven at 350 degrees Fahrenheit. Using a hand held mixer, combine all ingredients well, starting by creaming the butter, extracts and lemon zest together. Butter and flour the bottom only of a loaf pan and pour in batter. Gently tap loaf pan on a hard surface to remove air bubbles. Bake at 350 degrees for about 50 minutes or until a toothpick inserted into the center comes out clean. Once baked, let cool in loaf pan and sprinkle on confectioner sugar lightly on top.

Lilac Finger Sandwiches

1/2 Cup softened cream cheese
1/4 Cup lilac petals
1/4 Cup white sugar
1/2 teaspoon pure vanilla extract

Stir all ingredients together well with a wire whisk. Allow to chill in the refrigerator overnight. Spread on bread and use a cookie cutter to press out shapes and remove the outer crust. Brush on a bit of melted butter if you wish and then sprinkle on some purple granulated sugar. Perfect with tea at noon.

Hungarian Rose Fritters

All purpose white flour
Eggs
Spring water
1 teaspoon rose water extract (optional)
Whole milk
4 Tablespoons of white sugar
White or red roses

Exact measurements are not given because it all depends on the number of roses you have to prepare. Basically all you are doing is creating a dipping batter and coating the rose flower heads *only* with this batter. The battered rose is then placed in hot oil and fried until lightly golden brown, as you would for apple or pear fritters. Once cooled and allowed to drain on paper towels, sprinkle on the powdered sugar and enjoy!

Lavender Sugar Cookies

2 Cups all purpose white flower

3/4 Cup white sugar

4 Tablespoons finely ground lavender

2/3 Cup shortening

1 egg beaten

4 Tablespoon milk

1 teaspoon rose water extract (optional)

1 & 1/2 teaspoon baking powder

1/4 teaspoon salt

Preheat your oven to 375 degrees Fahrenheit. Cream shortening, sugar, extracts and lavender together well. Add egg and milk and whisk until fluffy and light. Stir in dry ingredients and combine well. Cover dough and chill in the refrigerator for at least 1 hour. Once chilled, pour dough out on a floured surface and roll out to a 1/8 thickness. Cut out shapes using cookie cutters and sprinkle with purple granulated sugar. Bake on an un-greased cookie sheet at 375 degrees for 8 to 10 minutes. Cool for 5 minutes on the cookie sheet and then remove to a cooling rack.

Rose Macaroons

The egg whites of 2 eggs

1/2 teaspoon of pure vanilla extract

1/4 teaspoon rose water extract (optional)

1 Cup finely chopped rose petals

2/3 Cup white sugar

1/4 teaspoon salt

Preheat oven to 325 degrees. With a wire whisk, beat egg whites, salt and extract(s) until soft peaks form. Gradually add in white sugar, continuing to whisk until stiff (and you're able to turn the bowl over with whites staying inside). Gently fold in rose petals. Use a teaspoon to drop lumps of cookie dough onto a greased cookie sheet. Bake slowly in a 325 degree oven for about 20 minutes. Let cool on a wire rack.

Rose Tea Sandwiches

1 stick of unsalted butter softened

1/2 Cup rose petals (or violet/clover)

1/4 teaspoon salt

In a small bowl, speed butter on the bottom and place a layer of rose petals over top. Cover petals with wax paper and the whole bowl with a lid or plastic wrap. Allow to stand in the refrigerator overnight or for 24 hours. After this time, remove all flower petals and add salt and a pinch of powdered sugar or honey. Combine well. Spread on white bread and trim edges of crust with a knife or by using decoratively shaped cookie cutters. What you are doing is infusing the butter with the delicious taste and scent of the roses or other flower type for a real treat. Instead of bread, slices of pound cake may be used as well.

Rose Syrup
1 Cup spring water
1 teaspoon rose water extract (optional)
1 Cup sugar
1 Cup fresh rose petals

Bring water to a boil and add extract and sugar. Stir constantly for 15 minutes and turn heat off. Promptly add rose petals and stir well. Allow to cool completely before pouring into a glass container. Very good on pancakes, buttermilk biscuits or ice cream. In India it is called Gulkhan and used on all sorts of confections and in mixed drinks.

Rose Jelly
1 & 1/2 Cups rose petals
1/2 spring water
1 & 1/2 Cups white grape juice
3 & 1/2 Cups white sugar
1 package of fruit pectin

Combine rose petals, water and grape juice in a sauce pan, bring to a rolling boil, being sure to stir constantly. Cook for 1 min. Add fruit pectin and sugar; cook stirring constantly, until mixture returns to a rolling boil. Continue boiling for 1 min. Remove from heat, and skim off foam. Quickly pour jelly into hot sterilized jar leaving 1/4 in headspace; cover with metal lids and screw tight. Process in boiling water bath for 5 minutes as you would for regular jellies. Allow to set in the refrigerator, which may take a few days. Very tasty on almost anything including sandwiches. Other floral jellies may be made in this manner as well including dandelion and violet. Be sure to remove any tart green portions of the flower, otherwise your jelly will take on a very unpleasant aftertaste.

Dinner Dishes:
Angelic Fish
2 pounds of flounder fillets
1/4 Cup chopped green onion
1/3 Cup angelica flowers

1/4 Cup butter

1/4 Cup finally chopped mushrooms

1 can of crab meat (save the liquid)

1/2 Cup salad croutons, crushed

1 teaspoon parsley

1/2 teaspoon salt

3 Tablespoons butter

1/4 teaspoon of salt

3 Tablespoons all purpose white flour

1/3 Cup white wine

1/2 teaspoon paprika

4 Tablespoon shredded Swiss cheese

Preheat oven to 400 degrees Fahrenheit. In a small pan, cook onion in butter until wilted. Stir in mushrooms and crab meat (save the liquid for latter), croutons, parsley, angelica, salt and pepper to taste. Place flounder into a non-greased baking dish. Spread the above *stuffing* mixture over fillets. Set aside. In a sauce pan, melt butter and blend in flour and salt. Pour crab meat liquid into a measuring glass and add enough milk to create 1 & 1/2 cups of liquid. Add this with wine to the butter/flour mixture and stir well. Cook and continue stirring until sauce is thickened and bubbly. This may take up to 15 minutes. Pour thickened sauce over fish and stuffing. Bake at 400 degrees for about 25 minutes. After this period of time, remove and sprinkle on paprika and Swiss cheese. Return fish to the oven and leave in for another 10 minutes or until cheese is brown and bubbly. Serve with fresh stemmed vegetables.

Honeysuckle Chicken

2 Cups cubed cooked chicken

3/4 Cup mayonnaise

1 Cup diced celery

1 Cup honeysuckle flowers

1 Tablespoon fresh lemon juice

2 Tablespoon diced green onion

4 Tablespoon Swiss cheese, shredded

Dash of salt

Preheat oven to 425 degrees. Combine all ingredients well and pour into a baking dish. Sprinkle on cheese over top and bake for 20 minutes or until cheese is golden brown and bubbly. If you will be cooking the chicken outdoors on a bar-b-q, you can actually burn the honeysuckle flowers on top of the coals for a delectable, sweet taste.

Dandelion Salad with Sunflower Bread

Salad:
1 Cup Lettuce
1 & 1/2 Cup dandelion greens
1/2 Cup dandelion flower heads
1 apple cubed
1 carrot grated
1/2 Cup borage flowers (optional)
Bread:
1 & 1/4 Cup bread flour
1/2 Cup wheat flower
1 Tablespoon milk powder
1/2 Cup sunflower petals
3/4 Cup spring water
1 Tablespoon butter
3 Tablespoon honey
3 Tablespoon sunflower seeds
1 & 1/4 yeast
1/2 teaspoon salt

Lightly wash greens and tea into smaller pieces. Toss all ingredients together and place in the refrigerator to chill.

Prepare bread according to bread machine directions for a regular loaf size. Remove bread and cut into 1/2 to 1 inch thick slices. Pile chilled salad on top of bread. Use a sweet vinaigrette if you like.

Rose Hip White Wine Soup
2 Cups spring water
2 Cups rose hips
1 teaspoon rose water extract (optional)
2 Tablespoon of cornstarch
1/2 Cup white sugar
1/2 Cup sweet white wine

To prepare this sweet soup, bring water to a boil and add rose hips. Cook until tender on very low heat, which is about an hour and a half of cooking time. In a separate bowl, combine cornstarch and sugar and add to the rose hip soup. Stir constantly until it begins to thicken. Once prepared, add white wine and cook for 5 more minutes. You may also wish to place hot soup in a blender for a few minutes to completely liquefy before serving.

· Chapter Seven ·

Floral Use in Homeopathy

The name Homeopathy is derived from the Greek words *homoios* meaning "similar" and *pathos* meaning "suffering". The main principle for the method of healing with Homeopathy is that "like cures like" and that by taking a remedy that mimics the actual symptom(s), the body will be stimulated to heal itself. Homeopathy is indicated for self limiting, chronic conditions that are not responding favorably to other forms of treatment or as a remedy for colds, fevers, flu, etc. The use of Homeopathic medicines was started by a German physician, Dr. Samuel Hahnemann 180 years ago. He was looking for a better alternative to the common practices of blood letting, the use of toxic substances such as mercury and came to the conclusion that certain botanicals, animal substances and minerals in a greatly diluted form had the power to aid the body in healing itself, naturally. He believed that the more diluted the remedy, the more potent it was. Substances that would be sometimes poisonous in normal doses, have the reverse effect on the body when taken in minute amounts, according to Homeopathic teachings. Much of the basis of Homeopathy is not to use the remedy to heal the condition but instead to bring on the symptoms further and cause the body to fight and combat the illness on its own, hence why remedies need to be taken over a extended period of time. There are many remedies on the market but we will be staying with those derived from flowering botanicals. As you will note, remedies are named after the substance's Latin name. This makes it easier to obtain and request remedies throughout the world as Latin names are universally known.

Homeopathic Flower Remedy Table:

Take either one of the remedies below only if you have the exact symptom. Remedies are not indicated to work unless the symptom or condition is matched with the particular Homeopathic medicine. There are 48 remedies in all but we will be staying with ones derived from flowering plants. By mixing remedies together, you can make special medicines to further aid in the healing process.

Bellis perennis (Daisy)—Bruises, Any sort of minor injury to the body, Aids in healing after surgery.

Calendula officinalis (Marigold)—Minor bleeding, Burns (first degree), Aids in healing after surgery, Sunburn, Break-outs of cold sores, Bed sores, Fungal infections.

Arnica montana (Arnica)—Bruises, Muscle and Joint pain, Over use of muscles-over exercising, Bad breath, Sprains, Pain associated with the back.

Chamomilla (Chamomile)—Colic, Asthma, Mild fevers, Earaches, Sleep problems, Gum irritation, Chronic skin conditions, Toothache, Teething and diarrhea in teething children, Carpel tunnel syndrome, Bed sores, Food poisoning (minor).

Gesemium sempervirens (Yellow Jasmine)—Anxiety, Over excitement, Fevers, Mild depression, Flu, Headaches, Heat prostration, Vertigo.

Hypericum perfoliatum (St. John's Wort)—Bruises, Minor wounds, HIV/AIDS, Minor head injuries, Insect bites.

Opium (White Poppy)—Digestion problems, Shock (emotional), Faintness.

Rumex crispus (Yellow Dock)—Teething, Coughs.

Pulstatilla nigricans (Pasque Flower)—Allergies-hey fever, Coughs, Chicken pox, Motion sickness, Shock (emotional), Ear infections, Anxiety, Mild depression-grief, Fevers, Faintness, Flu, Migraines, Sunstroke, Urinary tract problems, Mastitis, Teething, Vericose veins.

Symphytum (Comfrey)—Minor head injuries, Aids in the healing of broken bones.

Euphrasia (Eyebright)—Chills.

Aquilegia vulgaris (Columbine)—Nervous system problems.

How Homeopathic Medicines are Made

The botanical, animal tissue or mineral is ground into a very fine powder using a mortar and pestle. The powder is combined with 99 parts of ingestible alcohol and allowed to stand for a set period of time. One part of that mixture is combined with another 99 parts alcohol and the potency is then taken to another level. The resulting mixture holds an extremely tiny amount of original plant, animal or mineral substance, making it harmless and safe to ingest. Little sugar tablets are then medicated with the Homeopathic solution and placed in small containers. Mother solutions which are still providing that *one* part to be diluted with another set of successive 99 parts alcohol are sometimes over 100 years old. One arnica flower can yield thousands and thousands of bottles of Homeophatic remedies. It's not cost effective to attempt to make the remedies yourself. Buying them from a trustworthy company which has quality medicines is a better idea. Most of the time you will find them to be quite reasonably priced and contain a generous supply of pellets/tablets. Tables, pellets and liquid solutions come in dilution ratios which range from 1x that stands for 1 part substance to 9 parts dilution agency all the way to 200c that stands for 200 repetitions of diluting to 1 part substance with 99 parts dilution agency. Look for the higher ratios to be indicated with an "m," for a 1 to 999 ratio. Creams are also made out of Arnica and Calendula for external use.

How to Use Homeopathic Medicines Properly

Once you have found the medicine that most resembles your current symptoms, use them as follows.

-Before taking them make sure your mouth is free of other tastes. It is best not to take remedies within 30 minutes of any food, drinks, tobacco, vitamins, toothpaste or sweets.

-Homeopathic remedies should not be handled at all. Tablets, Pellets and granules should be tapped into the cap of the container and then given to or taken by the recipient. Some containers that the remedies come in have special tops that make this easy to do. Remedies should be placed directly under or on the tongue. A dose is generally three tablets. Don't swallow remedies but instead hold them in your mouth until they melt under the tongue completely.

-If you are using a Homeopathic tincture, make sure to hold the solution in your mouth for as long as possible. Don't simply swallow it.

-Babies and small children can aspirate the small pellets, tables, etc. Always dissolve the remedies in a spoon full of spring water before giving it to them or use a pre-made alcohol-free tincture.

-After you have taken the remedy, let it dissolve completely and do not take anything else, including more Homeopathic medicine by mouth for at least 20 minutes. This assures that the remedies has been completely absorbed into your system.

-If any remedies are spilled on any surface, dispose of them immediately. Never put them back into the container they came in. If you should touch the end of a liquid dropper, rinse it thoroughly before replacing it into the tincture bottle. Not doing so can lead to contamination of the medicines and loss of effectiveness. Oils from your hands, dust from surfaces, etc., all leads to the removal of the minute amount of remedy on each tablet.

-Do not stop any orthodox medication unless your medical physician approves of it. Homeopathy is not a replacement for medications and /or other methods prescribed to your by a health professional. If symptoms do not improve in a reasonable amount of time, seek medical attention by a medical physician.

How to Store Your Remedies

Just as with dried flowers, you must be quite careful with your Homeopathic remedies so that they do not lose their effectiveness.

-Keep remedies away from strong-smelling substances, i.e. perfumes, cleaning agents, paints and essential oils and also away from high temperatures and direct sunlight. Never attempt to transfer your remedies to another container. Always keep them in their original holder. If the container gets damaged by water or crushed, it's best to discard the whole thing and buy another bottle.

-If stored and handled correctly, homeopathic remedies should have no expiration date. It is recommend though, that remedies should be kept no longer than 2 years from the date of preparation which can be found on the bottle.

Using Homeopathy for healing is quite complex and revolves around the symptoms the person is experiencing. Careful watch must be taken and notes even as well to access and determine if the person is doing better or not. Doses are usually 3 tablets, pellets, etc. which are repeated over a certain period of time, i.e. every 3 hours, 6 hours, etc. Look on the backs of remedy bottles for recommendations. For exact dosages, you may want to seek the advice of a Homeophatic physician.

You will probably note that two of the most healing remedies are Arnica and Calendula which are flowers. They are indicated for many conditions and help with everyday problems and accidents. Most Homeopaths agree that no home should be without these two remedies.

· Chapter Eight ·
Floral Use in Kampo (Japanese Herbal Medicine)

Kempo is the 1,000 year old traditional herbal medicine of Japan and has strong roots from Traditional Chinese herbology and healing thought. Just as with Chinese medicine, Kempo uses cencepts to diagnose what a persons condition is. When these concepts fall out of balance, one will become ill. Cold and heat, excess and deficiency, interior and exterior along with yin and yang create the eight concepts or *Indicators* of Kampo medicine. As with most traditional forms of healing, Kempo is a holisticly based aproach to health and uses complex formulations of herbs to cure.

The largest part of Kempo is the actual diagnosing of conditions based on the indecators or symtoms one presents. Due to this fact, most people opt to only engage in Kempo under the direct care of a trained master Kempo herbalist or doctor. The doctor would attempt to detect any imbalances one has by symptoms they present including an over heated body, fever, red face, insomnia, etc., which are signs of a Heat/Cold imbalance. Once this is done, proper herbal formulations are prescribed. The doctor will also use 3 other forms of diagnosis borrowed from Chinese medicine, which is Blood, Fluid and the Vital Energy Qi. These body forces are also used to monitor a persons conditions and responce to the treatments.

As with Chinese medicine, teas are an important way of adminstering the herbal prescription, as are small herb filled capsills. In order for Kempo tea to work, it must be prepared very specifically to tradition. Metal pots or implements may not be used to make or hold the tea and water most be soft with a low minareal content. It must be boiled and simmered for at least 30 minutes and given in really condenced amounts and sticky gelatin like substances are also added to prevent herbs from berning at the bottom of the cooking pot. Herbs are not strained out like other tea preperations but instead ingested for further healing effect.

Just as with many forms of natural healing, flowers find there way into the healing preperations and Kempo is no diferent. A number of flowers have been traditionally used and are being included as Kempo spreads throughout the world. Below is a number of such floral botanicals and their traditional Japanese uses.

Kampo Herbal Chart

Byakushi or Wild Angelica—Used to help releave menstral and stomach problems.

Shukusha or Cardamom—Used mainly to improve Qi or live force, it also is used for chest pain, vomiting, constipation, etc.

Hokoei or Dandelion—Used to clear the liver, eye problems and for the stimulation of lactation in nursing women.

Kekketsu or Dracaena Lily—Used to dispel unmoving blood and heal bruses and contusions. Also applied to the skin and used in bone-setting.

Sanshishi or Gardenia— Used to control fevers and detoxify the blood.

Renshi or Lotus Seeds—Used to stop stress disorders including insomnia and anxiety.

Shini or Magnolia—Used to treat gastrointestinal problems and conditions related to "dampness".

Ozokukoku or Poppy (husk)—Used for giving lung Qi and to reduce pain of any sort. Also used for viral stomach conditions.

For the most part, Kempo does not use singular herbs but instead complex concoctions incorparating various ingredients including animal substances and minarals at times. These concoctions are then either powdered and placed in gelaten capsuls or turned into a tea elixir and prescribed for a number of weeks. In this period of time, monatering assures the pacent is recovering or not responding to treatment which leads to further assament or a change direction. Unlike Ayurvedic medicine which is based on ones whole lifestyle, Kempo is geared more twords painlessly adminstering prescribed herbal concoctions. The need for a change of diet or reduced consumption of alcohol was not an integrel part to the traditional Japanese medicine. Traditional Chinese alchemy advances would explain the basis for Kempo's aparent *magic pill* mentality.

Examples of Kempo Formulas:

Anchu-San:
Cardamom
Fennel seed
Cinnamon twig
Liorice

Oyster shell (powdered)

All ingredients would be powdered and given in pill form and would be used to build up energey in the body, concentrating on the middle section and all orgens in that region.

Senkyu-Chacho-San:
Angelica
Mint
Licorice
Pepperment

This formula is used to aid in the relief of headaches, dizziness, fever chils and other head cold type conditions. Traditionally, cold green tea is ingested along with this special blend to prevent side effects.

Today, Kempo is being incorparated with western medicine and other forms of holistic health which takes into considerations lifestyle also plays a role on ones overall health and changes need to be made along with the use of herbal concoctions at times.

· Chapter Nine ·

Floral Use in Ayurveda (Indian Herbal Medicine)

Ayurvedic medicine resembles both Chinese and Kempo Medicine as it is based on a life force, *Prana* or *ojas*, and five elements that may fall out of balance and cause illness. Earth, Air, Fire, Water and Ether make up these five important elements. Ayuvedic Medicine, which means "the science of life", is the oldest form of healing in India but was almost forgotten because of Mogul rularship and their own form of healing Unani Tibb which was adopted by the peoples from 908 to 1037 A.D. After Indian Independence, many returned to the ancient ways of Ayurvedic *living* which included Ayurveda in all aspects of ones life.

Ayurveda is a very holistic and complex form of healing which incorporates other aspects of diagnosis and healing including Chakras or "wheels" in Sanskrit and the 3 Doshas, *Prana, Agni* and *Soma*. Being that most Indian people are Vegetarians, Ayurveda is comprised mostly of healing with botanicals in dried herbal form and at times in essential oil form. Herbs are used to balance the forces in the body and help certain chakra areas of the body, which are associated with certain organs.

One of the easiest ways of using Aurvedic thinking and floral botanicals, is the chakra/essential oil connection. Chakra's in Aurvedic medicine are centers for body forces and today represent a section of the body and it's organs. There can be 8 to 12 chakras depending on cultural differences. Each chakra or wheel is associated with a special color which is used in color healing along with essential oil and herbal use. Similar to the Laws of Signatures, botanicals that are of the same specific chakra color may be used to treat associating organs and area of the body. Below is a chart of seven chakra's and their specific floral essential oils.

Chakra Essential Oil Chart

Crown Chakra (Magenta or White)—Associated with the pineal gland—nerolie, marigold

Brow Chakra or 3rd eye (Purple)—Associated with the pituitary gland—lavender

Throat Chakra (Blue)—Associated with the thyroid gland—blue chamomile, yarrow

Heart Chankra (Green)—Associated with the heart—rose

Solar Plexus Chakra (Yellow)—Associated with the liver—arnica, gardenia

Splenic Chakra (Orange)—Associated with the reproductive organs—tuberose, tagetes

Root Chakra (Red)—Associated with the reproductive organs—st. john's wort

You may also use this chart to create very special chakra perfumes or scents. Essential oils and herbs which have traditionally been used to aid in one of the associated organs would also be a fitting chakra botanical.

· Chapter Ten ·

Floral Use in Traditional Chinese Medicine

Traditional Chinese medicine, just like Ayurveda, is a very complex and holistic form of medicine as well as a very old form dating back to 2500 B.C.. Depending on the location of China you're at, there are many factors taken into consideration when Chinese doctors help their clients. Herbalisem is an integral part of the healing process and a number of the botanicals used are from flowering plants. Below is a list of such herbs and their Traditional Chinese uses.

Floral Chinese Herbal Chart

Shan zha (Hawthorn)—The berries are used to help stagnation problems including poor blood flow and digestion. In addition it is used for diarrhea problems.

Mo yao (Myrrh)—Used to heal wounds and to aid in blood circulation.

Chuan Xiong (Lovage)—Used to move Qi and the blood, it is used to reduce pain related to cold.

Qun Jiao (Gentian)—The roots are used to relieve digestion problems and feverish conditions.

Jin yin hua (Honeysuckle)—The buds are used to treat many conditions including fevers, diarrhea and dysentery.

Kuan dong hua (Coltsfoot)—The flowers are used for chest problems including asthma and bronchitis in addition to any coughs producing phlegm and decreased qi.

Jin ying zi (Rose)—The rose hips are primarily what is used in TC medicine. They are prescribed to help with the flow of qi or life energy and for urinary tract problems. They are also used for their astringent properties.

Pu gong ying (Dandelion)—The whole weed is used as a diuretic and liver function stimulant. Externally, it is used to heal skin abscesses and boils.

Zi hua di ding (Violet)—The whole plant is used for infectious skin conditions and for lymphatic system problems.

Zhi zi (Gardenia)—The fruit and roots are turned into a tea or tincture to detoxify the system and lessen fevers.

Hong Hua (Crocus)—Also known as saffron, in Traditional Chinese medicine, the safflower portion is used to move Qi and the blood along with relieving pain caused by poor circulation. *NOTE: Do not use if pregnant*

Like Ayurveda and Kempo, Traditional Chinese medicine also has principles which include the five elements, wood, fire, earth, metal and water, along with yin and yang an qi, life energy. Each one of these elements is associated with a number of body and earthly things including emotions, the seasons, colors, tastes, etc. Yin and yang on the other hand need to be balanced to maintain proper health. When they fall out of balance or qi levels are low, Chinese doctors attribute this to illness and use various forms of treatment including special massage and herbs to treat the conditions.

The main form of herbal prescription, is for special decoction teas to be taken for a number of days or weeks. These decoctions are much stronger than what westerns are used to drinking. About 100 to 200 grams of botanical to 1 liter of water is used and then reduced to about 300 milliliters or enough for 3 to 4 doses which can take up to 2 hours of cooking. At times, instead of whole dried botanicals, concentrated powders are created to be mixed with water to form tea. Herbs are also taken in capsule and natural pill form and combined together to create special treatments.

· Chapter Eleven ·

Floral Use In Native American Indian Medicine

Many wild flowers were used in Native American medicine in the forms or compresses, plasters, teas, etc., along with plants introduced by white settlers. In addition, many were also eaten on a regular basis. Far and away the most utilized all of flowers among Native Americans is the Purple Coneflower, more commonly known as Echinacea, (E. angustifolia). Used for everything from snake bite to colds and fever, Echinacea was used more than any other plant available by the indigenous tribes west of Ohio. The Sioux called this plant the "sacred herb" because its usefulness was beyond measure.

Although flowers were seldom gathered for their beauty as was commonly done by the settlers wives living on the prairie, flowers were left in their original growing areas because the native tribes felt that it was selfish to deprive others of their beauty when growing in the wild.

Perhaps the very most common edible flower of the indigenous tribes of the eastern woodlands was the sunflower. This plant is original to the United States as was gathered then as it is now for the highly nutritious seeds in the flowerhead. These seeds were often ground into a paste along with dried venison, berries and fat to form a highly concentrated food product called "pemmican". Sunflower seeds contain essential fatty acids, protein, vitamins and minerals and were taken on the trail by tribes while exploring and hunting. It was said that a bag of sunflower seeds and fresh spring water would sustain a brave for more than four days on the trail, maintaining his alertness and vigor. Today, many eat raw sunflower seeds for a great boost of natural energy in trail mixes and muffins. Then as now they are nature's powerhouse of energy.

Closely related to the sunflower is the Jerusalem Artichoke, also a Native American plant which was cultivated for food. Here the roots of this flower are tuberous and are prepared in a similar fashion to potatoes. The one health advantage of eating the Jerusalem Artichoke roots as opposed to white potatoes is that the Jerusalem Artichoke contains insulin. This substance is very beneficial especially for diabetics as insulin does not tax the pancreas the way sugar, (converted from the starch of potatoes), does. Today, many are tapping into the health benefits of the Jerusalem Artichoke by using breads and pastas made with this plant for health and superior nutrition.

Native American Medicinal Flower Chart

Fragrant Water Lily (*Nymphaea odorata*)—The root was turned into a tea for colds, mouth sores and bowl problems.

Prickly-Pear Cactus (*Opuntia humifusa*)—Used as a poultice to heal wounds and gout.

Common Evening Primrose (*Oenothera biennis*)—Root was used as a tea to treat bowl problems and obesity. Poultices were made to heal bruises and sore muscles.

Trout Lily (*Erythronium americanum*)—Root was used in tea form to reduce fevers and in poultice form to heal wounds and ulcers.

Passion Flower (*Passiflora incarnata*)—Poultices were used to heal cuts, boils and other skin afflictions.

Jerusalem Artichoke (*Helianthus tuberosus*)—Flowers were eaten or turned into tea to treat arthritis. Today the roots are turned into flour alternative food products.

Clover (*Trifolium repens*)—Used in tea form to reduce fevers and lesson cold symptoms.

Bluebeard Lily (*Clintonia borealis*)—Turned into a poultice to help heal cold sores, burns, rabid-animal bites, infections and bruises.

Common St. Johns Wort (*Hypericum perforatum*)—Flowers were used in tea form or as infused oil to heal ulcers, wounds, bruises as well as for depression and diarrhea.

· Chapter Twelve ·
Secret Flower Meanings
&
Victorian Charm

Before there were telephones and the moderately priced postage stamp, people would communicate through flowers. It is a known fact that people of the Victorian era were in love with flowers. Women would wear dozens of them in their hats and men would be frequently seen with a single flower on the lapel. Flowers were seen as much more then just pretty and fragrant. They were seen as symbols of emotions, thoughts and wishes. One of the common practices still seen today are birth flowers. Each month has its own flower and although it changes from place to place, I have found the following symbolism's pretty universal.

Birth Month Floral Chart
January: Carnation
February: Violet
March: Jonquil
April: Sweet Pea
May: Lily of the Valley
June: Rose
July: Larkspur
August: Gladiolus
September: Aster
October: Calendula
November: Chrysanthemum
December: Narcissus

It was thought to be quite auspicious for one to have flowers that were associated with their birth date to surround them in the home and work environment just as with birth stones.

Another popular thing to do in Victorian times was to use special floral containing pouches or sachets containing flowers and other amulets. The most common sort was one containing a love potion. These sachets were many times worn inside the dress of a woman at special events and gatherings. Other sorts of sachets were placed in bedding and clothing chests and closets to scent and protect the clothing as well as the wearer. Dried floral arrangements were also quite prevalent in the Victorian paler and household. Roses and other flowers were left on the steam, bundled and secured with a ribbon and left to dry. All were carefully prepared with special flower meanings attached.

Letter writing was also popular, mostly to the upper class as the postage stamp was quite expensive at that time. Another item was the calling card which was like a modern day business card. When people came calling for the lady or gentleman of the house and they were unavailable, the visitor would leave their calling card in a special candy dish like respectable. These cards for lavishly decorated or quite plane depending on the class of the holder. Stationary, calling cards, greeting cards, etc. were kept in pretty boxes that were filled with aromatic flowers, mainly lavender. We know today that lavender is very calming, soothing and anti-depressing. It also helps the immune system to fight sickness.

Complete List of Flower Meanings Table:

The following is a list of flower meanings which I have found to be pretty universal all over the world. Next time you give the gift of fresh or dried flowers, give a hidden, ancient meaning or wish as well. Some of the meanings were coined in Victorian times while others were started in far away countries thousands years ago. Many believe that the secret flower language started in Constantinople in the 1600s and was brought to England in 1716 by Lady Mary Wortley Montagu who had spent time in Turkey with her husband. The interest quickly then moved to France, which was the capital of the perfume industry, where the Book Le Langage des Fleurs was printed with over 800 floral signs and meanings. The English translation of Book Le Langage des Fleurs at the time of Queen Victoria was toned down a bit because some of the meanings were thought to be too risqué for Victorian readers.

Le Langage des Fleurs Chart

A

Alastruemeria ....Intrigue
Apple blossom ....Preference
Aster ....Memories

Azalea ....Temperance
B
Begonia.......................Deformity
Buttercup ....Childness
C
Calendula ....Grief, Despair,Sorrows
Carnation ....Refusal,
Chamomile................Energy in hard times
Chrysanthemum........Love, Friendship,Truth
Clover........................Be mine, Think of me
Cowslip ....Divine beauty
Crocus ....Abuse not
D
Daffodil ....Regards
Daisy ....Innocence, Beauty
Dandelion..................Loves oracle
Delphinium ....Ardent Attachment
F
Forget-me-not...........True love
Freesia.......................Trust
G
Gardenia....................Untold love
Geranium ....Comfort
Gladiolus ....Strength of character
Golden-rod...............Be cautious
H
Heliotrope ....Devotion
Hibiscus ....Delicate beauty
Honeysuckle..............Devoted affection
Hyacinth...................Sorrowful
Hyssop ....Cleanliness
J
Jasmine.....................Grace & Elegance, Joy
Jonquil ....Affection
L
Larkspur ....Lightness
Lavender...................Distrust
Liatris ....Gladness
Lilac ....Youthful innocence

Lily ....Purity, Sweetness
Lily of the Valley ....Return of happiness, Purity
Lotus ....Mystery, Truth, Estranged love
M
Magnolia ....Love of nature
Marigold....................Jealousy
N
Narcissus....................Egotism, Precious moments
O
Orange blossom ....Chastity
Orchid ....Beauty
P
Pansy ....Thoughts
Passion flower ....Faith
Periwinkle..................New friendship
Peach blossom............Captive love
Pink ....Boldness, Refusal
Poppy, red..................Consolation
Poppy, white ....Sleep
Primrose ....Sadness
Q
Queen Anne's Lace ....Haven
R
Rose ....Love, Devotion, Beauty
Rose, cabbage ....Ambassador of love
Rosemary ....Remembrance
S
Snapdragon................Intrigue
Sweet Pea ....Love, Departure, Delicate pleasures
T
Tulip.........................Hopeless love
Thyme ....Courage
V
Verbena......................Pray for me
Violet ....Modesty, Steadfastness
Z
Zannia ....Thoughts of absent friends
Secret Language of Roses

Roses also have a secret meaning of their own, depending on their color and size. Keep this in mind before sending a dozen to a loved one.

Pale pink....................Purity, Lovely grace, Sweetness
Red............................Respect, True love
Deep pink..................Love, Beauty
Peach ....Modesty
Deep red....................Bashful shame, Love
Orange ....Passionate fascination and love
Yellow........................Jealousy, Friendship
White ....Worthiness of your love, Fear
Blue ....Uniqueness
Burgundy ....Unconscious love
Single Pink Rose bud Simplicity
Thornless ....Fresh attachment, Love

Victorian Recipes

Victorian's were in love with flowers, especially roses and exotic varaties with spicey scents. Pot-pourrie was one of the most popular forms of scenting a room and were placed everywhere from the palor to bowls placed on the stove filled with hot water. Below are a few traditional recipes and their many applications.

English Rose Blend
1/2 Cup roses
1/2 Cup orange flowers
1/2 Cup lavender
1/2 Cup jasmine
1 Tablespoon thyme
1 Tablespoon sage
1 Tablespoon marjoram
1 Tablespoon bay
3 Cups rock salt
10 drops sandalwood essential oil
1 teaspoon oriss root
4 Tablespoons cassia flowers
1 cinnamon stick
2 Tablespoon whole cloves
1/4 teaspoon benzoin gum
10 drops rose essential oil
2 drops musk fragrance oil
1/2 Tablespoon crushed cardamine seeds

Place all ingredients into a large earthenware or glass bowl and combine well. Cover with a tight fitting lid or plastic wrap and allow to cure for a few weeks, in a dark, dry enviornment. Any dampness may result in mold growth which will ruin your pot-pourri. After it has cured, use it any way you wish!

Simple Floral Blend

3 Cups rose petals

1 Cup lavender

2 vanilla bean pods

1 Tablespoon oriss root

5 drops each of rose and lavender essential oil

Combine all ingredients well and store in a container with a lid or a plastic bag for 1 week to cure. Be sure to store it in a dry, dark place so mold will not effect it. Once cured, use it as you like. The vanilla pods may be broken up into smaller pieces to release more of their scent as time goes on.

Pot-pourrie Wreath

Using a pre-made wreath base which could be made out of Styrofoam or a natural substance such has hay or vines, glue pot-pourri to the base using white or hot glue. Let it cure completely overnight before proceeding with the embellishments. This will make sure the pot-pourri doesn't droop or fall off. Once cured, gently use wire to hold the wreath together and then wrapped lightly with ribbon. The ribbon is simply for show and doesn't need to be secured like the wire. If you find the scent of the wreath has greatly diminished, don't throw it away. Instead, re-scent it by spraying it lightly with essential oils mixed with a few teaspoons of water.

Variation:

Instead of using a wreath base, you can use a ball shape, most frequently done in Styrofoam and coat it entirely in white glue. Roll the ball in a bowl of pot-pourri and allow to dry completely overnight on a bed of newspaper. These balls can then be hung from ribbons and placed decoratively in a bowl. These balls were very popular in Victorian times, displayed on a wooden stick in a flower pot to depict a small tree.

Boxed Pot-pourri

This fun project is very simple and can use a varity of sized boxes. The most important item needed to make this project work, is a netting or screan material. You can use a fabric material which is very gauze like or a section from an old window screan made of wire. This will allow air to flow through the box and the wonderful scent of pot-pourri to escape but not the plant material itself. Cut a whole, smaller than the piece of netting material you have, in the lid of the box. Completely wrap with decorative paper, fabric or do a special painted finish, to the outside of the box. From the inside, glue the piece of netting and allow to dry overnight. Fill with desired pot-pourri blend and tie lid down using a ribbon. These boxes are lovely when stacked together on a coffee table or placed in each one of your closets to lightly scent belongings.

· Chapter Thirteen ·
Flowers Garden

Growing flowers yourself can not only be an extremly rewarding experience but also a wonderful hobby. When you grow your own flowers, you can be in full control of what is sprayed or applied to them. This is especially important when you will be using your flowers to create concoctions or for cooking. In addition, you can be sure the soil you are using is organic as well and rich in nutrients which will be carried into the growing plant. Below you will find helpful insight into controling pests naturally and growing a better flower garden organically through special recipes and techniques I personally use on my own flowering plants.

Flower Planting Chart

Flowering Plants that Like Full Sun

Marshmallow

Borage

Feverfew

Marigold

Soapwort

Thyme

Comfrey

Mustard

Chamomile

Sunflower

Rose

Muskmallow

Hyssop

Lavender

Poppies

Evening Primrose

Geraniums

Flowering Plants that Like Light Shade

Sweet Rocket
Honeysuckle
Soapwort
Muskmallow
Bee Balm
Rose
Violet
Nasturtium
Flowers that Climb
Roses (look for climbing verities)
Honeysuckle
Begonia
Clematis
Jasmine
Nasturtium
Passionflower
Trumpet Vine
Vetch
Wisteria
Flowers that Aid Other Plants

Certain flowers, when planted along side other plants will actually work with each other to repel pests and grow better. People in the horticultural field are looking into the way plants might be able to communicate to one other through their root systems, growing healthier than plants grown in a single, non-harmonies environment. The following is a short list of these such varieties.

Nasturtium:

Plant near any plant to help repel aphids. It seems to attract a fly, hoverflies, that attack aphids on the nasturtium itself and nearby plants. Makes a good companion to almost any herb, vegetable, berry plant.

Thyme:

It can be planted anywhere you need to control bean beetles, cabbage butterflies, root flys, and carrot flys. Tends to spread and take over so keep confined to small areas of your garden.

Lavender:

Helps repel mosquitoes, moths of various types, black flys and fleas which works well if your flowers are planted near a back porch, patty-o or deck. Lavender grows well when planted next to nasturtiums and foxglove.

Marigold:

This is one of the most common plants used for repelling pests. Use as a border flower for the perimeter of your garden to help reduce white fly and eel worm damage. Some also say the roots of the plants repell moles and mole rats.

Natural Pest Control

Reaching for a spray bottle of pesticide to douse your flowers with is not a good idea if you are planning to use your flowers for medicinal or culinary purposes. This is one of the biggest reasons you are growing your own flowers, to protect yourself and love ones from pesticides, hormones, radiation, etc., which can come with non or even organically grown herbs and dried flowers. Along with planting certain flowers next to each other, also known as companion planting, here are a few natural pest controls you can prepare using everyday, household items.

Rose Spray

5 Cups water

5 to 10 (depending on size) cloves of garlic

2 to 3 teaspoons powdered garlic

5 drops essential oil of hyssop or 4 to 5 tablespoons dried hyssop

Bring water to a boil and add garlic cloves, hyssop (if dried) and powdered garlic. Turn heat off and let stand 1 to 2 hours. Remove from the stove once cooled and place in a blender or food processor. Blend until liquefied. Strain off any plant material and empty liquid into a spray bottle. Mist effected plants a couple of times a day. This will make your flowers smell of garlic but the alternative of damage by aphids and other pests is worse in certain cases. Rain will was away the odor after a while. To intensify the effects of this treatment even more, add freshly ground black pepper to the boiling water before adding garlic. When I didn't have any fresh garlic on hand, I was able to use just the powdered cooking garlic with success as well.

Sun Teas for Plants

3 to 5 Cups water

Dried or fresh thyme, hyssop, rosemary or lavender

2 to 3 drops essential oil(s) of the above (optional)

Place the plant material into a clear mason jar and add water. Let sit in the sun for a week or longer as with any other sun tea. Instead of pouring the tea directly on plants or roots, which can cause damage, dilute 1/4 cup in another 4 cups of water. Use to spray plants to help control pests.

Variations:

Essential oils can be used in place of dried or fresh repellent flowers. Simply add up to 10 drops of essential oil into 1 gallon of water. For more concentrated formulas, use less water to dilute the essential oil. This works well if you want to make a natural pest control spray right on the spot and not have to wait for it to cure like a sun tea. Be careful that you do not damage your plant with concentrated essential oils applied directly to the plant or roots. Never use fragrance oils in place of essential oils.

Powders can be made by using dried, powdered orris root and adding essential oils and powdered herbs. Be sure to mix your powder well and let it cure for a few days. You want the orris root to absorb the pest control benefits of the added essential oils or herbs. To apply, simple sprinkle over effected areas. Watch for signs of continued damage. If you see any, you might need to take more drastic measures.

Chamomile Tea

Make a simple tea decoction of chamomile flowers and water, letting it steep for 5 minutes. Let cool completely before pouring over plants. Make sure it gets down into the root system. This will help prevent and clear up mold. Works especially well on seedlings which are prone to mold damage.

Lady Bugs

Many organic gardeners view the lady bug as a dear friend. They do a lot to control harmful pests on a large scale outdoors. They are many times found naturally in the wild but if you find their numbers too low in your garden, you can simply buy some from a nursery or mail order catalog. To help persuade them to stay in your garden, spray the leaves of your plants with a simple solution of molasses and water. To combine the ingredients well use a food processor or blender. Doing so will not harm your plants and will also help to attract bees for pollination.

Store/Nursery Bought Plants

The most important thing to do if you buy large plants from a nursery, store, etc., is to make sure there are no signs of bug infestation. Most plants with aphids and other pests are usually not that healthy to begin with. Look for drooping and discolored leaves as an indication. After checking the plant over for pests, make sure there is no mold, fungus or blight on the leaves, steams or flowers. Flowering plants with holes eaten away in the petals should also be avoided even if the bugs are not found. Before you plant the plants in your garden or set it along with your other plants, give it a bath on a bowl of water and pest repelling essential oils. To do this, leave the plant in it's pot and turn it over, dipping the top of the plant in the water/essential oil solution. Dunk for a few seconds and lift out. Set plant in the sun to prevent mold or mildew. Not only does this clean the plants leaves but it also help kill bugs that you might have missed.

· Afterword ·

This book actually has it's own story of how it became. The author, Marie Anakee, got the idea of writing a book that would document and bring all of the interesting medicinal history flowers have in one place. Through much research and use of her own personal experimentation, How Flowers Heal became a reality in early 1998. A major Park Ave. New York publisher immediately sent a contract for publishing the book in a full color, coffee table version. Not what Marie Anakee originally had in mind for her book, she went ahead and formatted the book as set forth by the publisher. The publisher did not have stock pictures for the book or a photographer for the over 150 illustrations needed and placed the burden of this on Ms. Miczak with the stipulation they would reimburse the photographer. After seeing the very low amount of money they were willing to pay, she desided to ask her brother, international photographer J.Y. Miczak who's pictures have appeared in books, magazines and the web to do the job. Together Marie and Joe visited many botanical gardens in and about New Jersey to take slides of specific flowers including "2 Deep Cut Gardens" in Middletown which was a lovely trip. Johnny Selected Seeds was also kind enough to donate slides from their catalog for inclusion in the book. When all was said and done, over 150 slides were taken with few duplicates. This took months to complete and in this time, even though the contracts were sent back way ahead of starting the project, no advance or reimbursement was ever sent. The publisher also failed to send back signed copies of the contract to Marie Anakee as they said they would in the letter that accompanied contracts. The Acquisitions editor had no qualms about calling though with questions on how the project was going and complaining the slides were not cropped properly which wasn't even the job of the photographer. Physically and monetarily drained, Marie Anakee decided she would halt work on the book for this publisher until the signed contracts were returned to her and the advance paid. She of course heard nothing from the publisher and received no money.

Marie Anakee still had the dream that her book would be published but could no longer work on it full time. She set it aside and started work on her 3rd book, "Mehndi: Rediscovering Henna Body Art". At the start of 1999, the original contract from the New York publisher had expired; but in reality had been broken by the publisher long before by their not paying the advance in "a few weeks" as they stated they would. Marie Anakee was still working on her 3rd book when the publisher called a few months later acting if nothing out of the norm had happened and explaining they had found a photographer for the book and very much wanted to proceed. In complete disgust, she never returned their calls and vowed to finish "How Flowers Heal" how she originally envisioned it, filled with wonderful recipes and interesting medicinl content. A few months later the book was finished and is how you read it now. This book is the result of not only many hours of writing and researching but driving to botanical gardens to get a first hand look at every botanical mentioned here, interviewing experts, contacting companies, growing the flowers in her own organic garden, testing the recipes and finding informative articles to include. The result is a highly unique volume that the author hopes you not only treasure but use often and find comfort in. If you would like to learn more about the author and her latest books and/or contact her, please visit http://www.miczak.com .

· About the Author ·

Marie Anakee Miczak has been trained as an Aromatherapist and has studied herbology and the culinary arts. In addition to this book, she is the author of "Secret Potions Elixirs & Concoctions: Botanical & Aromatic Recipes for Mind, Body & Soul" (Lotus Press) and "Mehndi: Rediscovering Henna Body Art" (BBOTW). She has taught related courses at Brookdale College NJ and is Contributing Editor for Aromatherapy at Suite101. A prolific writer, Ms. Miczak appears frequently in magazines, newspapers and other publications off and on the web. She lives with her faimly and dog in NJ where one of her favorite pastimes is evening flower gardening.

· Appendix ·

Resource List

Essential oils:
(Remember, the higest quality essential oil needs to be used for a productive outcome. Using low grade essential oils is many times just as bad as using Fragrance oils and will lead to a waste of money and time. Look for companies that sell professional "Aromatherapy" grade essential oils which are steam distilled and preferably organic.)

Aromatherapeutix
phone: 1-800-308-6284
FAX: 562-795-0002
3062 Kumpton Drive
Los Anamitos, CA 90720 USA
Very nice selection of pure essential oils for all your Aromatherapy needs.

Aroma Vera
phone: 1-800-669-9514
web: http://www.aromavera.com
Known for their very high quality essential oils. Frequently used by professional Aromatherapists.

Natural Skin Care Products:

Brookside Soap, Inc.
phone: 206-742-2265
FAX: 206-355-6644
P.O. Box 55638
Seattle, WA 98155 USA
web: http://www.halcyon.com/brookside/
e-mail: BrooksideSoap@msn.com

A wonderful selection of herbal soaps, bath soaks/salts, bath oils and massage oils. If you haven't the time to make your own right that second, they are a wonderful alternative!

Incense Products:

Inciendo De Santa Fe, Inc.
phone: 505-345-0701
320 Headingly Avenue North West
Albuquerque, NM 87107 USA
Incense and burners made from aromatic wood and botanicals from the American South West and Native peoples living there. My personal favorite is the Victorian bath tub complete with bubble bath lid incense burner.

Perfume Bottles:

Gazelle Glass, Inc.
phone: 514-929-6464
FAX: 541-929-4364
31364 Peterson Road
Philomath, OR 97370 USA
web: http://www.proaxis.com/~gazelle
e-mail: gazelle@proaxis.com
Hand-blown glass bottles to hold all of your perfume blends.

Herbs:

Herb Products Company
phone: 1-800-877-3104
11012 Magnolia Boulevard
P.O. Box 898
North Hollywood, CA 91603-0898 USA
Large selection of quality dried herbs. Especially useful as tea and for herbal blending.

Seeds/Plants:

Johnny's Selected Seeds
phone: 207-437-9294

Fross Hill Road
Albion, ME 04910 USA
web: http://www.johnnyseeds.com
e-mail: staff@johnnyseeds.com
Renowned for their selection of organic seeds and plants for starting your own garden. Large selection of flowering herbs to pick from as well. They also give tours from July to August, daily at their 24 acre Main USA location. A wonderful company!

Schools

Kevala—IYS
Hunsdon Road
Torquay
Devon, TQ1 1QB England
web: http://www.kevala.co.uk
e-mail: info@kevala.co.uk
Very well done, international home study courses in Aromatherapy and other related alternative health studies. One of the few Aromatherapy schools to be accredited and require case studies to be done prior to graduation.

· Notes ·

Quick Medicinal Flower Reference

Arnica: Arnica montana

Also known as: Leopard's Bane

Origins: Asia, Europe

Healing effects: Works to help heal bruises and soreness when in a cream form. Researchers are looking into the way it might stimulate the immune system to keep one from coming down with colds and flu.

Warnings: Never use on open cuts or broken skin. The flowers of the plant are toxic and should only be used in cream or homeopathic form.

Bee Balm: Monarda didyma

Also known as: Wild Bergamot

Origins: North America Healing effects: Very healing, it can be infused to form a tonic tea and to help stop nausea and sleep problems. Using it in a steam bath or sauna can help colds, coughs and sore throats.

Bergamot (see Bee Balm).

Betony: Stachys officinalis

Also known as: Bishopswort

Origins: Europe

Healing effects: Helps to promote circulation to the brain, calm nerves and heal minor wounds. It has a long history of use dating back to ancient Egypt and Rome. May be taken in tincture, poultice or infusion form.

Borage: Borago officinalis

Also known as: Star flower

Origins: Europe

Healing effects: The flowers and leaves are edible, smelling of cucumber they can be turned into a tea to help relieve depression and stress. The leaves contain many vitamins and minerals including potassium.

Warnings: Over indulgence in borage leaves or flowers can cause side effects including stomach and bowl discomfort. Do not over use.

Boronia: Boronia megastigma

Also known as: Brown Boronia

Origins: Australia

Healing effects: This plant is many times grown ornamentally in small gardens. It is mostly used for its aromatic flowers and expensive essential oil which can be used in perfumes.

Cactus Flowers: Cactus grandiflorus
Origins: Americas
Healing effects: The plants, used fresh and made into a tonic/tea that may help heart, kidney and bladder problems.
Warnings: Use only in moderation.

Coltsfoot: Tussilago farfara
Also known as: Horse Hoof
Origins: Asia
Healing effects: May be turned into a decoction or infusion to treat asthma, coughs and other respiratory problems.
Warnings: Some say it has carcinogenic attributes and should no longer be used medicinally and have been banned in some countries.

Comfrey: Symphytum officinale
Also known as: Knitbone
Origins: Europe
Healing effects: Contains many minerals and vitamins that help in cell regeneration and growth which is especially helpful for broken bones and bruises. A poultice can be made from the leaves and placed over swollen joints or areas to alleviate the pain and help reduce the swollen area. The same cell rejuvenating qualities can also work on aging or sun damaged skin.
Warnings: Use only in moderation internally. Research as noted liver damage in laboratory animals who were given high doses and as a result it has been banned in some countries.

Cornflower: Centaurea cyanus
Also known as: Bachelor's Button
Origins: Found many places
Healing effects: An infusion can be prepared and used as a hair and skin tonic and treatment. A tea can also be made for use for indigestion.

Cowslip: Primula veris
Also known as: Paigle
Origins: Europe, Asia
An edible flower which is used for candied flowers and cake decorations, it is also used as a flavoring for foods and wine. Use as a decoction for chronic skin conditions such as acne and to help reduce fine lines. A tea can be made of the flowers to help calm and relieve stress along with sleep problems. Best if taken before bed.

Warnings: May cause contact dermatitis to people with sensitive skin. Do a patch test before using. Being that it is sedative, do not ingest if you plan on operating machinery of any kind.

Daisy, English: Bellis perennis

Also known as: Lawn Daisy

Origins: Europe, Asia

Healing effects: May be used as a infusion for external use to help bring life back to dull skin and to help relieve chronic skin conditions such as acne and eczema.

Warnings: Certain people may find it causes allergies, do a patch test before use.

Heliotrope: Heliotropium spp.

Also known as: Cherry Pie, Turnsole

Origins: Rainforests of Peru

Healing effects: This flower which is used in the perfume industry for its wonderful scent, was used by the Incas to reduce fevers. Mostly used for its aromatic qualities which help to calm nerves.

Warnings: Use in moderation.

Hollyhock: Althaea rosea

Also know as: Blue or Purple Malva

Origins: Europe, Asia

Healing effects: Related to the marshmallow plant/flower, hollyhock's were used in cosmetics to help heal damaged skin. Infusions were made for use as a tonic.

Iris: Iris pallida

Also known as: Orris root

Origins: Mediterranean

Healing effects: The root is used in powder form as a natural fixative and preservative. The powdered root can also be used as a body powder base and for hair treatments.

Warnings: Use in moderation.

Lady's Smock: Cardamine pratensis

Also known as: Cuckoo Flower

Origins: Europe

Healing effects: Contains a good amount of vitamin C and was traditionally used to help cure scurvy. It also has mild expectorant qualities and works well in a cough syrup form for administration.

Lilac: Syringa vulgaris

Also known as: Syringa

Origins: Europe

Healing effects: Mostly used for its aromatic qualities, lilac comes in 3 main colors of white, pink and the traditional purple.

Lily of the Valley: Convallaria majalis
Also known as: May Lily
Origins: Europe, North East Asia
Healing effects: Mostly used for its aromatic qualities it was turned into a tonic decoction tp strengthen the heart and relieve water retention. It is thought of as a safer form of Digitalis, as it contains many of the same attributes but in a weaker form.
Warnings: Plant is toxic and should only be used by educated physicians. Fragrance oil of plant may be used like any other aromatic ingredient.
Lotus: Nymphaea lotus
Also known as: Many names depending on local
Origins: Found many places
Healing effects: Used mostly in the perfume industry for its lovely scent. Depending on variety , the juice was used to heal chronic skin conditions and as a tonic.
Warnings: The lotus mentioned has toxic tubers and should not be ingested.
Neroli: Citrus aurantium
Also known as: Orange Flower
Origins: Far East
Healing effects: Scent is said to be hypnotic and help one to sleep. Calms nervous disorders and is an anti-depressant as well.
Warnings: Use externally only, in essential oil form.
Pansy: Viola tricolor
Also known as: Heartsease
Origins: Europe
Healing effects: Fresh flowers may be used in an ointment or salve for minor skin conditions to promote healing. A decoction can also be made, traditionally for STD's. The flowers and plant were also used to help heal rheumatism and gout.
Periwinkle: Vinca major
Also known as: Sorcerer's Violet
Origins: France, Italy
Healing effects: Traditionally used for stopping bleeding and toothaches. Also used on minor wounds to promote faster healing.
Soapweed (see Yucca)
Soapwort: Saponaria officinalis
Also known as: Bouncing Bet
Origins: Europe, Asia

Healing effects: When added to water or made into a decoction the plant softens the water and makes a gentile wash for hair, skin with chronic conditions such as acne, etc. as well as old delicate clothing and rugs.

Warnings: The root of the soapwort is toxic so use externally only.

Sunflower: Helianthus annuus

Also known as: Chimalati

Origins: Americas

Healing effects: The fresh or dried seeds of the sunflower may be eaten as a snack which will intern provide many important B vitamins. The oil is quite healing and can be used as a base oil in Aromatherapy and message blends.

Sweet Rocket: Hesperis matronalis

Also known as:

Origins: Italy

Healing effects: Traditionally used for treating and preventing scurvy. It is quite aromatic and the flowers may be used in culinary dishes.

Warnings: Large doses may cause nausea, consume in moderation.

Ylang Ylang: Cananga odorata

Also known as: Unona odorantissimum

Origins: Malaysia, Philippines

Healing effects: Used mostly for it's aromatic oils in perfume and Aromatherapy applications. It has a stimulating and anti-depressing effect on the body.

Yucca: Viburnum opulus

Also known as: Soapweed, Needle Palm

Origins: America

Healing effects: Yucca has been used by native people of south eastern United States for thousands of years for food and for personal care. The root may be used in a salve or poultice for healing sores and to help relieve sore muscles.

Articles on Medicinal Use of Flowers

Below is a collection of articles previously published at www.suite101.com by their respective authors. I hope you enjoy reading them as much as I did.

Drive-By Echinacea

by Barbara M. Martin

Have you seen it? Maybe not a showstopper, but an eye-catcher nonetheless. Plant identification at 60 plus miles an hour on a winding road through the Ozarks is always a treat, but when you are driving at the same time it can be a bit of a challenge. What, I thought, is *that*? I squinted at a tall skinny plant leaning into the sunlight on a blind curve. A skimpy sort of coneflower. Prominent cone, stringy limp petals hanging down and curving inward, definitely purple but washed out and pale. Bingo! Pallor is the key. Echinacea pallida right there in real life. Cousin to the E. purpurea garden variety purple coneflower. Known to herbalists forever. Native to North America. And striking in its own way, growing like a ghost on the edge of a limestone cliff. I'd know it anywhere now that I've seen it, and so might you if you are a prairie fan or if you are into medicinal herbs. Many of us know and grow its relative the purple coneflower (Echinacea purpurea) as a high performance, long-blooming and showy perennial valued not just for its beauty, but also for its amazing power to draw butterflies and its virtually unstoppable ability to laugh at extremes of heat and cold and drought. Many of us have noticed myriad herbal remedies touting "echinacea" as a panacean ingredient, too. (E. angustifolia is another variety you may see listed on a label.) Some might almost consider echinacea to be a household word once again in this "new" age of natural remedies and herbal healing. But how well do we know or standardize our ingredients ? Do you know which of the coneflowers is the endangered species ? And maybe most intriguing of all is to trace this plant's recorded history from Native American knowledge through today's modern commercial crop production practices and then we can only begin to guess at its future as science unravels the mysteries of nature. Ready to add some coneflowers, purple or otherwise,to your garden? Check out this excellent quick Overview, Culture and Uses http://www.egregore.com/herb/echinacea.html page and find out about~Echinacea Species here http://www.islandnet.com/eclectic/species.html.-Originally published at Suite101.com.

Angelica: The Angel of Herbs

The Angel of Herbs
by Karyn Siegel-Maier

If you have ever stood next to an herb that was taller than you (or the first story of your house), it was probably angelica. The fact that it can reach up to 8 feet in height would make calling the herb "tall" an understatement indeed.

There is some confusion though as to how angelica (*Angelica archangelica*) received its reverent name. Some say that it was so named because it reputedly blooms on May 8th of each year, the day of the feast of the Archangel St. Michael. Others believe it's name was bestowed by a monk who either had a dream or vision in which the Archangel Raphael appeared and pronounced the herb to be a cure for the scourge of the mid-17th century—the plague. Perhaps for this reason, angelica has been a long-standing favorite herb in pagan healing rituals, offering magical powers of protection. Medicinally, angelica has a long list of ailments it has been used to cure. You'll recall that Raphael presented angelica as a cure for the plague. Well, it's curative powers must have been impressive, for angelica water became a primary constituent of the formula published by the College of Physicians in London. Known as the "King's Majesty's Excellent Recipe for the Plague," the formula combined angelica water, treacle and nutmeg. The brew was simmered over a fire and given to plague victims twice each day.

Angelica was generally revered as a health restorative as it could allegedly add years to one's life. The roots were used to make Carmelite water, a tonic that was taken to ward off evil spirits and to ensure long life. In 1974, French journalists wrote about Annibal Camoux of Marseilles upon her departure from this world and offered the conclusion that she had lived to the ripe age of 120 because she had chewed angelica root every day.

Angelica was also incorporated into brews to treat rabies, digestive disorders and as an eye and ear wash to "help dimness of sight and deafness." Medieval monks made preparations from the root for lung disorders, such as pleurisy, asthma and bronchitis. Native Americans used angelica to treat tuberculosis and consumption. As a poultice, angelica was applied to bruises and inflammatory conditions. Modern herbalists recommend angelica to regulate the menstrual cycle. A relative of angelica known as don quai (*A. sinensis*), is well known for its use in gynecology and obstetrics, as well as for its ability to improve liver function impaired by hepatitis or cirrhosis. Angelica was equally at home in the kitchen. Its use as a flavoring has been known since the Vikings introduced the herb to Europe in the 10th century. The candied stems were once a popular confection and they were the green candies in the first fruit cakes. Norwegian cooks relish the flavor the powdered root lends to baked goods. Benedictine monks used angelica to flavor wines, and it is still an ingredient in vermouth, gin and Chartreuse.

Traditional Candied Angelica

This takes a bit of effort, but you'll have fun making these candies. Children really enjoy this project as well.—Warning: Don't harvest angelica from the wild since it has been mistaken for a hemlock that grows in the same environment. It's best to obtain the stalks from your own garden, or a reputable nursery.

2 cups angelica stems (the young shoots) 2 cups boiling water ½ cup salt Syrup: 2 cups sugar 2 cups water 1 tbls. lemon juice Put the angelica in a large bowl and cover with the salt and boiling water. Cover with a tea towel and let stand for one full day. Then drain, peel and rinse the angelica in cook running water. To make the syrup, cook the sugar and water to the syrup stage on a candy thermometer, about 240'F. Add the angelica and lemon juice and cook another 20 minutes, stirring often. Drain off the angelica stems, reserving the syrup. Refrigerate syrup and place the angelica on a rack and store in a cool, dark place (like a pantry or cupboard) for 3-4 days. Return the syrup and angelica to a pot and cook about 15-20 minutes or until candied. Drain angelica and store on a rack until thoroughly dry. Store in a covered jar or container.-Originally published at Suite101.com.

Dance of the Violets

by Karyn Siegel-Maier
"That which above all others yields the sweetest smell in the air, is the violet..."—*FrancisBacon*

As a distinguished member of the Violaceae family, the violet (*Viola spp.*) shares it's roots with few relatives. In fact, its only cousins are pansies and garden violas. While the genus *Viola* numbers more than 500 in species, the number of hybrid varieties probably outnumber the pure ones. Much loved by various cultures throughout the world, the essential violet, *Viola odorata*, has been widely cultivated for more than 2,000 years. This highly aromatic and ornamental herb has enjoyed a long association with romance, fertility, and occasions for joyous celebration. The Romans welcomed the arrival of spring by scattering violet petals and leaves in banquet halls and with the partaking of *Violetum*, a sweet wine formulated by the gourmet Apicius.

The ancient Greeks made the violet the official symbol of Athens. Legend has it that Zeus protected his lover, the goddess Io, from the jealous Hera by turning his love into a heifer and allowing her to graze unseen upon a meadow of sweet violets. In 13th century France, troubadours were bestowed with great cascades of violets in appreciation of their poetic achievements. Napole`on Bonaparte made the violet his "signature flower." It became the emblem of his political party, and a symbol of everlasting love between he and his first wife, Josephine.

Josephine reputedly honored her husband by scattering violet petals on his final resting place.

Medicinally, the violet has been employed to remedy a variety of ailments. The Romans believed wearing a band of violets about the head would ensure sobriety during festivals and would deter "morning after" unpleasantness. (One wonders if this prevention arose out of necessity from the habitual imbibing of too much violet wine!) Preparations formulated from violets to ease hangover pangs are still popular in France today. Pliny recommended violet water for gout and spleen disorders. The leaves and flowers are reputed to have an expectorant quality and "Violet Plate," a violet sugar or conserve, was a popular ingredient in 17th century throat lozenges and cough syrups. For centuries, violets have been used to treat fever and headache, and in China today to treat abscesses and as a poultice for inflammation. The results were likely effective since the plant contains an aspirin-like substance known as methyl salicylate. The flowers are still used today to tint certain medications.

Victorian nosegays and "strewing" potpourri of the 18th century usually included violets due to their soporific effect. Although fresh violets are highly fragrant when first cut, their very scent, as well as undesirable odors that may be present at the time, become less noticeable very quickly. Shakespeare's Laertes made reference to this mysterious quality when he said: *"A violet in the youth of primy nature, Forward, not permanent; sweet, not lasting. The perfume and suppliance of a minute. No more."* Great quantities of the sweet violets are commercially grown in France and Italy today for the perfume industry. It takes more than 2 million flowers to produce a single pound of the essential oil! A low-growing perennial reaching approximately 4 inches in height, the violet is particularly suitable for rock gardens, banks, as a border for ponds or anywhere groundcover is desired. It will prosper if given a moist, rich bed of soil of between 7 and 8 pH and plenty of sun, although most varieties will tolerate partial shade. Violets can be easily transplanted to your garden from the wild as long as you are able to duplicate the conditions in which it was found. Since violets grow on runners, they will spread rapidly each year and may need thinning out. Also, the flower heads will burst forth with more frequency if excess runners are trimmed.

The violet is quite agreeable to propagation by seed or root division, but the easiest method is to clip the off-shoots in early spring and root them in soil at least 1 foot apart. Some species can be grown from seed sown in outdoor frames in early autumn, the seeds of which need to experience freezing temperatures before they will germinate. However, the frames should be covered with burlap until germination occurs, usually within 10 to 20 days. Cover the frames with mulch to protect the young plants from winter's chill. The flowers of different species of violets range in color, but most frequently they are deep purple, blue, white, or pink. The pansy, or *V. Triclor* is one of the more popular hybrids due to its particularly beautiful flowers. Several species are native to North America, such as *V. Blanda* and *V. Lanceolata*, both of which are aromatic and thrive in swampy conditions. *V. Pedata* is prized for it's large flowers which reminds one of a bird's foot. This species produces flowers of every conceivable color. Other popular species are *V. Palmata*, which makes an early entrance in late winter; *V. sagittata*, the leaves of which grow to an unusually large size after flowering; and *V. rostrata*, which enjoys a moist, rocky environment. *V. pubescens* produces large pale green foliage and the flowers of *V. rotundifolia* are an exquisite yellow. The Canadian violet, *V. Canadensis*, is an unusually tall species that yields white star-shaped flowers. Most violets have slightly toothed leaves of varying degree and shape which is probably why what is commonly called the dog-tooth violet is often mistaken as a relative. The association ends with the common name since the dog-tooth violet, or *Erythronium denscanis*, is actually a member of the Liliaceae family. Similarly, although several species of violets are to be found in Africa, the African violet (*Saintpaulia ionantha*) is not related to the true violet. Violets may be somewhat inconspicuous singularly, but will very soon take over whatever space is afforded to them and they will continue to delight you with sprays of color for many seasons. There is another reason to celebrate the appearance of violets other than the arrival of another growing season, and for the same reason you'll want to have an abundance of flower heads available. They're great fun to prepare and serve in salads, jams, soups, puddings or even as the old fashioned crystallized treat. Bon Appetite!

Violet Custard

This is a simple but elegant dessert, or you can serve it at brunch. It's equally good warm or chilled. It's especially attractive because the violets float to the top! 3/4 cup violet petals 3 large eggs 2 egg yolks 1/2 cup sugar 3 cups milk 1 tsp. Vanilla Divide the violet petals between 8 individual ramekins. Beat together the eggs, yolks, and sugar. Blend in the milk, vanilla, and sugar. Divide the custard among the ramekins and place them into a large baking dish. Add enough boiling water to the large baking dish to reach the halfway point on the ramekins. Place the baking dish with ramekins in the oven, lower the temperature to 325' F, and bake for 45-50 minutes. The custard is done when a knife inserted in the center comes out almost clean.-Originally published at Suite101.com.

The Chamomiles

by Karyn Siegel-Maier

"How the Doctor's brow should smile Crown'd with wreath of camomile…"
—Thomas Moore Wreaths for the Ministers

While many people recognize the name chamomile (or camomile, an alternate spelling), few actually realize that two different species share the same name. Both possess the same medicinal properties and fragrance but have clear differences. Roman chamomile *(Chamaemelum nobile)* rarely reaches a foot in height and renders a bitter flavor. It was once a very popular groundcover for English lawns. German chamomile is the species likely to be found in herbal teas, medicinals and cosmetic preparations.

Although the chamomiles bear no resemblance to the fruit in any way, they were called *kamai melon* (to mean ground apple) by the ancient Greeks who favored their apple-like fragrance. The Spanish referred to chamomile as *mazania*, or "little apple," and used them to flavor their finest sherry. Inspired by chamomile's medicinal value, the Germans described it as *alles zutraut*, or "capable of anything." Chamomile (German) has long been used to ease tension, indigestion and headache. You may recall that Peter Rabbit's mother nurtured his aching head with chamomile tea after he'd had a night of indulging in Farmer McGregor's garden. Chamomile was also a popular remedy for muscle pain and menstrual cramps. In fact, the Romans rubbed the herb on sore muscles and sprains. Taken internally, chamomile does seem to have an anti-inflammatory action. A clinical study published in the Journal of Clinical Pharmacology in 1973 on the anti-inflammatory qualities of chamomile produced some interesting results. Ten out of twelve subjects who were given chamomile tea reportedly dozed off to sleep within ten minutes, even while they were undergoing a painful procedure. (Personally, I'm not very likely to rely upon chamomile at the moment of a tooth extraction, but I would highly recommend it for muscle soreness and headache.) The therapeutic benefits of chamomile are due to the presence of *chamazulene*, bisabololoxides A and B and matricin. The flower heads contain quercimertrin, apigenin and luteolin (flavonoids) which also lend anti-spasmotic and anti-infammatory qualities, as well as the coumarins herniarin and umbelliferone. Chamomile may be an old-fashioned remedy, but more than 4,000 tons is cultivated and harvested each year world-wide.

A word of caution is warranted in the use of chamomile by allergy sufferers. The chamomiles (sometimes including yarrow) do contain some degree of allergens. Only 50 cases of allergic reaction have been reported between 1887 and

1982, however, with five of these being a direct result of consuming German chamomile. Still, it would be advisable to avoid frequent use of chamomile if you are known to be sensitive to chrysanthemums or ragweed.-Originally published at Suite101.com.

How Essential Oils are Produced

by Marie Anakee Miczak

The extraction process of essential oils has a long and interesting history, believed to have started in ancient Egypt and further discovered in the days of the Alchemist. Here we will take a deeper look into how essential oils are extracted today and how these various methods shape the resulting oils effectiveness, quality and usability. One thing that should be pointed out from the start, is essential Aromatherapy grade oils are extracted from once living botanical sources including flowers, fruits, barks and even resins from trees. Many commercial institutions wishing to jump on what they see as a craze for Aromatherapy "like" products, blur the lines as to what essential oil use really is and would like you to believe that fragrance oils may be used in the essential oils place, being just as effective. The truth of the matter is, there are actually two branches which have become intertwined, mainly by the perfume industry. The art of Aromatherapy is not simply inhaling pleasing essential oils for mood enhancement, an aphrodisiac effect, etc., this falls more into the realm of Aromacology, which is the study of scents and fragrances on the human psyche and mind. Aromatherapy on the other hand is the use of highly concentrated essential oils which not only have an effect on the psyche from it's aroma but also medicinal qualities which can be used in a variety of applications including inhalation, massaging on the skin, cold and hot compresses, etc. Aromacology may use non-real alcohol based perfumes while Aromatherapy can only use pure, real essential oils. Here is a look at the various ways of extraction which is used today.

Infused oil AKA Maceration: Base oils such as vegetable or sweet almond are mixed with aromatic plants, the mixture is heated over a fire or placed in the sun.

Distillation: Plant material is placed inside a still like contraption. Steam is forced passed through the botanicals like an espresso maker. The essential oil filled pockets in the botanical burst open and the essential oil is carried away as the steam travels to the top of the still. The steam is forced into a water-cooled pipe (condenser) where the vapors return to a liquefied state. Essential oils float to the top of the water and are spined off. The water that remains is used as floral waters.

Enfleurage: Lard is smoothed over a large glass plate. Flower petals (such as rose) is then spread on top of the lard. This is done over and over until the lard has absorbed the oils and scent of the flowers. Alcohol is used to remove the essence of the flowers from the lard. The remaining lard is used in soap making.

Expression: Citrus fruits such as limes, lemons, oranges, etc. are peeled and the zest is used and pressed (such as with apple cider) to remove the oils. The oils collect into sponges which are later squeezed to produce the finished product of essential oils. This method while completely natural and very desirable is not used as often as solvent or steam distillation.

Solvent Extraction: Hydrocarbon solvents are used in a drum filled with plant material to dissolve the essential oils. The solution is filtered and put through a distillation process. It produced resinod and concrete. Alcohol is used to extract the oils and the finished product is called an absolute. Unfortunately not all the solvents or alcohol can be completely removed and the resulting essential oils, which can result in a less effective product.

Carbon Dioxide: Carbon Dioxide gas or butane is used when in a liquefied state to extract oils from plants under extreme pressure. This is a very new development in essential oil extraction methods and is still under testing and modification. Once again, as with the solvent method, this procedure may lead to denaturing of the essential oil and it's effectiveness.

One of the best and oldest methods of obtaining essential oils and not denaturing them or add impurities is distillation. Alchemist were known for their use of distilled botanicals and believed that everything, including stones, sand, etc., could be distilled to produce healing medicines. A large potion of their thinking that anything earthly could hold healing properties, was the belief that everything had a soul and spirit which could be extracted and used by the human body, referred to as "solve and coagula". The Alchemists art of "spagyrie" was to distill the botanical over and over again to remove all impurities and produce what they thought to be a highly potent and powerful medicine. At the turn of the century in France the distillation process could only be done on a small scale, mainly for wild lavender. Today it is still successfully used for the extraction of essential oils and preferred by Aromatherapists far and wide. Many botanicals, especially flowers produce a very small yield of essential oil for the volume of petals picked. This has of course made these certain essential oils more costly to produce and to buy, by the consumer. Factors such as this has lead to the use of mock essential oils more and more by companies and the fragrance industry. While saving a few dollars may seem good at the time it can mean you are not going to get the results you are looking for or even a allergic reaction from the chemicals used. Always read the label carefully to see what is inside the bottle. It should only be the plant used for the extraction and perhaps a base oil such as jojoba, peanut or sweet almond.

Some companies are now producing organic essential oils. Any pesticides or chemicals on the plant can end up in the essential oil, so organic oils make very good sense. The fragrance industry makes a point of always brining up that essential oils can not be standardized and that everyone should use chemical reproductions which are always the same instead. People said that herbs couldn't be standardized either yet now we see many companies including pharmaceutical ones producing such products. There are far too many components that essential oils contain for there to be an exact chemical match made of them. The first area and most important to the perfume industry to be copied is the scent and not the other components which include vitamins and nutrients. I'm sure it will be a matter of time before standardized essential oils are also produced. by MAM-Originally published at Suite101.com.

Note: A very old form of essential oil extraction from India is making a comback. Attars, mainly used as perfume, is the steam distillation (think pressure cooker) of flowers in a base of sandalwood essential oil. Instead of using a base oil such as neem, all attars are rendered in low grade sandalwood oil. Through the high pressure distillation, the scent of the sandalwood is displaced by the scent of botanical extracted. The resulting essential oil Attar is highly concentrated. Some people are attempting to use Attars in Aromatherapy settings. Due to the sandalwood base, these Attars may be unsuitable for Aromatherapy use as even though the scent has been displaced, it does not mean the principal constituents have been which may lead to denaturing of final products.

Buy These Other Titles by the Miczak's

Nature's Weeds, Native Medicine: Native American Herbal Secrets (Lotus Press) by Dr. Marie Miczak, Ph.D
ISBN: 0-914955-48-9

-Nature's Weeds, Native Medicine offers a unique insight to the secret healing herbs used by the first inhabitants of North America.-

To order, please call toll free 1-800-824-6396 or visit Amazon.com.

Secret Potions, Elixirs & Concoctions: Aromatic & Botanical Recipes for Mind, Body & Soul (Lotus Press)

by Marie Anakee Miczak
ISBN: 0-914955-45-4

-This interesting book contains, in an easy-to-understand form, many ways to utilize botanicals including essential oils, herbs and more for use in everyday life.-

To order, please call toll free 1-800-824-6396 or visit Borders.com.

Mehndi: Rediscovering Henna Body Art (BBOTW)

by Marie Anakee Miczak

ISBN: 0-7414-0280-7

-This immensely interesting book contains, in practical and easy to understand form, every detail on creating fantastic Mehndi designs using natural henna.-

To order, please call toll free 1-877-BUYBOOK or visit BN.com.

For a complete list of Miczak Books, please visit http://www.miczak.com or e-mail drmiczak@myhost.com .

· Glossary ·

Allergy:
Reaction caused by what the body perceives as a foreign substance.
Anemia:
Deficiency of iron containing red blood cells, which causes sleepiness, fatigue, low body temperature, etc.
Annual:
Plants that grow from a seed, flowers, and dies in one season. These plants don't always return the next season like perennials and bulbs.
Antibiotic:
Destroys or stops the growth of bacteria.
Antidepressant:
May help to relieve the symptoms of depression and lift the spirits.
Antiseptic:
Destroys or helps to prevent the growth of microbes.
Antiviral:
Helps to prevent the growth of viruses.
Aphrodisiac:
Induces amour or stimulates desire for another person.
Arthritis:
Inflammation of the tissue surrounding the joints of the body which causes pain.
Aromatherapy:
The use of pure essential oils for healing of the soul and body.
Aromatic:
Pleasing aroma that is used in perfume or to scent the environment.
Biennial:
A plant that has a life cycle of two years. Usually growing to produce leaves, stems, root system, etc. the first year and flowers, seeds, fruit, etc. the next and dying there after.
Bronchitis:
Inflammation of the bronchi of the lunges.
Capsule:

A small, empty pill made of gelatin which can be filled with powdered flowers for ingestion.

Cellulite:
A dimpled appearance under the skin, mostly affecting women.

Deciduous:
Plants that drop their leaves at the end of each growing season.

Deodorant:
A substance that covers over or removes unpleasant smells and odors.

Digestive:
Substance that promotes or helps in the digestion of food, drinks, etc.

Diuretic:
A chemical agent that stimulates the bladder to expel excess water in the bodies system as well as toxins.

Disinfectant:
Helps prevent the spread of germs.

Emollient:
Aids in softening and smoothing the other layers of the skin.

Enflerage:
The extraction of aromatics from flowers by the method of using fats such as lard. Used for many years, it is no longer cost effective and is only done on a small scale now.

Expectorant:
Substance that aids in the removal of mucus and phlegm from the lunges and respiratory system.

Fixative:
A substance that helps reduce evaporation of volatile oils and aids in keeping aromas in perfumes, potpourris, etc.

Fungicidal:
Helps prevent and kill fungus.

Genus:
Group of similar plants that are cauterized to be in the same family.

Herbaceous:
Usually a perennial plant that doesn't have woody steams which dies down at the end of the growing season.

Hybrid:
A plant which has been altered by man or out in nature forming a new subspecies.

Menopause:
The stopping of menstruation later in a woman's life.

Sedative:

A substance that induces sleep.

Synergy:

Two substances are used together for a heightened effect on the system.

Shrub:

A perennial which has branches for stems that are woody and which doesn't grow more than a few feet high.

Species:

Classification given to a plant within a genus for identification.

Tonic:

A herbal concoction for healing the whole body.

Topical:

Application of a substance to the outer body, such as the skin and hair.

PMS:

Premenstrual syndrome. A condition categorized by water retention, moodiness, etc.

· References ·

Aromatherapy

Jeanne Rose & Susan Earle (Editors), *The World of Aromatherapy* (Berkeley Califonia: Frog Ltd. 1996)

Julia Lawless, *The Illustrated Encyclopedia of Essential Oils: The Complete Guide to the Use of Oils in Aromatherapy and Herbalism* (Shaftesbury Dorset: Element Books 1995)

_____, *Secret Potions, Elixirs & Concoctions: Botanical & Aromatic Recipes for Mind, Body & Soul* (Twin Lakes, WI: Lotus Press 1999)

Valerie Ann Worwood, *The Complete Book of Essential Oils & Aromatherapy: Over 600 Natural, Non-toxic & Fragrant Recipes to Create Health, Beauty, A Safe Home Eviornment* (San Rafael, Califonia: New World Library 1991)

Kempo

Robet Rister, *Japanese Herbal Medicine: The Healing Art of Kempo* (Garden City Park, New York: Avery Publishing Group, Inc. 1999)

Herbology

Lesley Bremness, *Herbs: The visual guide to more than 700 herbs species from around the world* (London: DK 1994)

Michael Castleman, *The Healing Herbs: The Ultimate Guide to the Curative Power of Nature's Medicines* (Emmaus, PA: Rodale Press 1991)

Penelope Ody, *The Complete Medicinal Herbal: A practical guide to the healing properties of herbs,with more than 250 remedies for common ailments* (London: DK 1993)

Native American Herbology

Marie Miczak, D.Sc., Ph.D., *Nature's Weeds, Native Medicine: Native American Herbal Secrets* (Twin Lakes, WI: Lotus Press 1999)

Steven Foster/James A. Duke, *Eastern/Central Medicinal Plants* (Peterson Field Guides) (New York, NY: Houghton Mifflin Company 1990)

Ayurveda

Miriam Polunin and Christopher Robbins, *The Natural Pharmacy: An illustrated guide to natural medicine* (New York, NY: Collier Books [DK] 1992)

Chinese Medicine

Stefan Chmelik, *Chinese Herbal Secrets: The Key To Total Health* (Lewes, East Sussex: The Ivy Press Ltd. 1999)

· Bibliography ·

botanical.com—A very interesting site, it contains the entire 1940's book "A Modern Herbal" by Mrs. Grieve, F.R.H.S.

Miczak.com—Visit for all sorts of interesting and informative articles by the Miczak's on a number of topics including Aromatherapy, safe herbal use and much more. The official website of Marie Anakee Miczak.

_____. *Secret Potions, Elixirs & Concoctions: Botanical & Aromatic Recipes for Mind, Body & Soul* (Lotus Press: 1999)

Philip B., *Blended Beauty: Botanical Secrets for Body & Soul* (Ten Speed Press: 1995)

Suite101.com—Visit the Wellness and Gardening areas for some wonderful topics ranging from roses to natural health, traditional Chinese medicine to herb gardening. Each topic has a Contributing Editor, most of the time an expert, to answer your questions, write in-depth articles and find the best links on the net. Be sure to visit my Aromatherapy area at http://www.suite101.com/welcome.cfm/aromatherapy .

Index

A

Arnica; 1-2, 5, 18, 66-68, 74, 99, 123
Ayurveda; 0, 73, 75-76, 119, 123

B

Bee balm (see Bergamot); 2, 8, 33, 58, 88, 99, 123
Bergamot; 8, 17, 24-25, 27, 99, 123
Borage; 1, 10, 33, 58, 64, 87, 99, 123
Box, Pot-pourrie; 123

C

Calendula; 1, 10, 20, 23, 49, 52-53, 55, 58-59, 66-68, 79, 81, 123-124
Chamomile; 1-2, 6, 17, 23-24, 27, 33, 36, 51-56, 58, 66, 74, 81, 87, 90,
        109-110, 123
Clove pink; 6, 123
Clover, Red; 123
Columbine; 66, 123

D

Daisy, Lawn; 123
Dandelion; 1-2, 10, 43, 58, 62-64, 70, 75, 81, 123
Dog rose (see rose); 123

E

Eucalyptus; 24, 54-55, 123
Evening primrose (see primrose); 2, 78, 87, 123

F

Feverfew; 1-2, 10-11, 33, 87, 123
Forget me not; 12, 123

G

Gardenia; 9, 17-18, 27-29, 58, 70, 74, 76, 81, 123
Geranium; 1-3, 17-18, 23, 27-28, 33, 45, 47, 57, 59, 81, 123

V

Violet; 1-3, 14, 17-18, 27-29, 33, 42-43, 46, 51, 59, 61-62, 76, 79, 82, 88, 102, 106-108, 124

W

Wild Passion Flower; 13, 124

Y

Yarrow; 2, 14, 23, 36, 74, 109, 125
Yucca; 4, 59, 102-103, 125